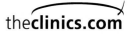

UROLOGIC CLINICS
OF NORTH AMERICA

Urologic Imaging

GUEST EDITOR
Pat Fox Fulgham, MD

CONSULTING EDITOR
Martin I. Resnick, MD

August 2006 • Volume 33 • Number 3

SAUNDERS

An Imprint of Elsevier, Inc.
PHILADELPHIA   LONDON   TORONTO   MONTREAL   SYDNEY   TOKYO

W.B. SAUNDERS COMPANY

A Division of Elsevier Inc.

1600 John F. Kennedy Boulevard • Suite 1800 • Philadelphia, Pennsylvania 19103-2899

http://www.theclinics.com

UROLOGIC CLINICS OF NORTH AMERICA Volume 33, Number 3
August 2006 ISSN 0094-0143
Editor: Kerry Holland ISBN 1-4160-3919-8

Urologic Clinics of North America (ISSN 0094-0143) is published quarterly by Elsevier Inc., 360 Park Avenue South, New York, NY 10010-1710. Months of issue are February, May, August, and November. Business and Editorial Offices: 1600 John F. Kennedy Blvd., Suite 1800, Philadelphia, PA 19103-2899. Customer Service Office: 6277 Sea Harbor Drive, Orlando, FL 32887-4800. Periodicals postage paid at New York, NY and additional mailing offices. Subscription prices are $210.00 per year (US individuals), $325.00 per year (US institutions), $240.00 per year (Canadian individuals), $390.00 per year (Canadian institutions), $280.00 per year (foreign individuals), and $390.00 per year (foreign institutions). Foreign air speed delivery is included in all *Clinics* subscription prices. All prices are subject to change without notice. **POSTMASTER:** Send address changes to *Urologic Clinics of North America*, Elsevier Periodicals Customer Service, 6277 Sea Harbor Drive, Orlando, FL 32887-4800. **Customer Service: 1-800-654-2452 (US). From outside the US, call 1-407-345-4000.**

Urologic Clinics of North America is covered in *Index Medicus*, *Excerpta Medica*, *Current Contents/Clinical Medicine*, *Science Citation Index*, and *ISI/BIOMED*.

Printed in the United States of America.

CONSULTING EDITOR

MARTIN I. RESNICK, MD, Lester Persky Professor and Chairman, Department of Urology, Case Western Reserve University, School of Medicine/University Hospitals, Cleveland, Ohio

GUEST EDITOR

PAT FOX FULGHAM, MD, Urology Clinics of North Texas, Dallas, Texas

CONTRIBUTORS

GILAD E. AMIEL, MD, Baylor Prostate Center, Scott Department of Urology, Baylor College of Medicine, Houston, Texas

J. KYLE ANDERSON, MD, Department of Urology, The University of Minnesota; The Veterans Affairs Medical Center, Minneapolis, Minnesota

MATTHEW J. BASSIGNANI, MD, Associate Professor and Section Chief, Genitourinary Imaging, Department of Radiology, University of Virginia Health Sciences Center, Charlottesville, Virginia

TIMOTHY J. BRADFORD, MD, Resident, Department of Urology, University of Michigan Medical Center, Ann Arbor, Michigan

JEFFREY A. CADEDDU, MD, Department of Urology, The University of Texas Southwestern Medical Center, Dallas, Texas

ROBERT S. DAVIS, MD, Department of Urology, University of Rochester Medical Center, Rochester, New York

VIKRAM DOGRA, MD, Associate Chair of Education and Research, Director of Ultrasound, Director of Radiology Residency, Professor of Radiology, University of Rochester School of Medicine, Department of Imaging Sciences, Rochester, New York

C. RICHARD GOLDFARB, MD, Chief, Nuclear Medicine Division, Department of Radiology, Beth Israel Medical Center, New York, New York

DRAGAN J. GOLIJANIN, MD, Department of Urology, University of Rochester Medical Center, Rochester, New York

AARON B. GROTAS, MD, Department of Urology, Beth Israel Medical Center, New York, New York

KHALED S. HAFEZ, MD, Assistant Professor, Department of Urology, University of Michigan Medical Center, Ann Arbor, Michigan

JASON T. JANKOWSKI, MD, Resident, Department of Urology, Case Western Reserve University, MetroHealth Medical Center, Cleveland, Ohio

FADI N. JOUDI, MD, Fellow Associate, Department of Urology, University of Iowa, Iowa City, Iowa

DAVID M. KUEHN, MD, Assistant Professor, Department of Radiology, University of Iowa, Iowa City, Iowa

CHARLES G. MARGUET, MD, The Comprehensive Kidney Stone Center, The Division of Urology, Department of Surgery, Duke University Medical Center, Durham, North Carolina

JAMES E. MONTIE, MD, Valassis Professor of Urologic Oncology and Chairman, Department of Urology, University of Michigan Medical Center, Ann Arbor, Michigan

HARRIS M. NAGLER, MD, Chief, Department of Urology, Beth Israel Medical Center, New York, New York

FUKIAT ONGSENG, MD, Department of Radiology, Beth Israel Medical Center, New York, New York

LANE S. PALMER, MD, Chief, Pediatric Urology, Schneider Children's Hospital of the North Shore-Long Island Jewish Health System, New Hyde Park, New York; Associate Clinical Professor, Departments of Urology and Pediatrics, Albert Einstein College of Medicine, Bronx, New York

SANGTAE PARK, MD, MPH, Acting Assistant Professor, Department of Urology, University of Washington School of Medicine, Seattle, Washington

MARGARET S. PEARLE, MD, PhD, Professor of Urology and Internal Medicine, The University of Texas Southwestern Medical Center, Dallas, Texas

GLENN M. PREMINGER, MD, The Comprehensive Kidney Stone Center, The Division of Urology, Department of Surgery, Duke University Medical Center, Durham, North Carolina

W. BRUCE SHINGLETON, MD, Department of Urology, The Lousiana State University Health Sciences Center, Shreveport, Louisiana

ERIC A. SINGER, MD, MA, Department of Urology, University of Rochester Medical Center, Rochester, New York

KEVIN M. SLAWIN, MD, Baylor Prostate Center, Scott Department of Urology, Baylor College of Medicine, Houston, Texas

J. PATRICK SPIRNAK, MD, Professor, Department of Urology, Case Western Reserve University and Director, MetroHealth Medical Center, Cleveland, Ohio

W. PATRICK SPRINGHART, MD, The Comprehensive Kidney Stone Center, The Division of Urology, Department of Surgery, Duke University Medical Center, Durham, North Carolina

NEIL C. SRIVASTAVA, MD, Department of Radiology, Beth Israel Medical Center, New York, New York

RICHARD D. WILLIAMS, MD, Professor and Head, Rubin H. Flocks Chair, Department of Urology, University of Iowa, Iowa City, Iowa

CONTENTS

Selection and application of appropriate imaging modalities for patients undergoing percutaneous nephrostolithotomy enhances the safety and success of the procedure.

GOAL STATEMENT

The goal of *Urologic Clinics of North America* is to keep practicing urologists and urology residents up to date with current clinical practice in urology by providing timely articles reviewing the state of the art in patient care.

ACCREDITATION

The Urologic Clinics of North America is planned and implemented in accordance with the Essential Areas and Polices of the Accreditation Council for Continuing Medical Education (ACCME) through the joint sponsorship of the University of Virginia School of Medicine and Elsevier. The University of Virginia School of Medicine is accredited by the ACCME to provide continuing medical education for physicians.

The University of Virginia School of Medicine designates this educational activity for a maximum of 15 AMA PRA Category 1 Credits™. Physicians should only claim credit commensurate with the extent of their participation in the activity.

The American Medical Association has determined that physicians not licensed in the US who participate in this CME activity are eligible for 15 AMA PRA Category 1 Credits™.

Category 1 credit can be earned by reading the text material, taking the CME examination online at http://www.theclinics.com/home/cme, and completing the evaluation. After taking the test, you will be required to review any and all incorrect answers. Following completion of the test and evaluation, your credit will be awarded and you may print your certificate.

FACULTY DISCLOSURE/CONFLICT OF INTEREST

The University of Virginia School of Medicine, as an ACCME accredited provider, endorses and strives to comply with the Accreditation Council for Continuing Medical Education (ACCME) Standards of Commercial Support, Commonwealth of Virginia statutes, University of Virginia policies and procedures, and associated federal and private regulations and guidelines on the need for disclosure and monitoring of proprietary and financial interests that may effect the scientific integrity and balance of content delivered in continuing medical education activities under our auspices.

The University of Virginia School of Medicine requires that all CME activities accredited through this institutions be developed independently and be scientifically rigorous, balanced and objective in the presentation/discussion of its content, theories and practices.

All authors/editors participating in an accredited CME activity are expected to disclose to the readers relevant financial relationships with commercial entities occurring within the past 12 months (such as grants or research support, employee, consultant, stock holder, member of speakers bureau, etc.). The University of Virginia School of Medicine will employ appropriate mechanisms to resolve potential conflicts of interest to maintain the standards of fair and balanced education to the reader. Questions about specific strategies can be directed to the Office of Continuing Medical Education, University of Virginia School of Medicine, Charlottesville, Virginia.

The authors/editors listed below have identified no professional or financial affiliations for themselves or their spouse/partner:

Gilad E. Amiel, MD; J. Kyle Anderson, MD; Matthew Bassignani, MD; Catherine Bewick, Acquisitions Editor; Timothy J. Bradford, MD; Jeffrey A. Cadeddu, MD; Robert S. Davis, MD; Vikram Dogra, MD; Pat Fox Fulgham, MD; C. Richard Goldfarb, MD; Aaron B. Grotas, MD; Khaled S. Hafez, MD; Jason T. Jankowski, MD; David M. Kuehn, MD; Charles G. Marguet, MD; Fukiat Ongseng, MD; Lane S. Palmer, MD, FACS, FAAP; Sangtae Park, MD, MPH; Margaret S. Pearle, MD, PHD; Martin I. Resnick, MD; Eric A. Singer, MD, MA; Kevin M. Slawin, MD; J. Patrick Spirnak, MD; W. Patrick Springhart, MD; Neil C. Srivastava, MD; Alon Z. Weizer, MD

The authors/editors listed below identified the following professional or financial affiliations for themselves or their spouse/partner:

Dragan Goliijanin, MD holds a patent with Novadaq Technologies, Inc.
Fadi N. Joudi, MD, FRCSC has a research project sponsored by Gyrus ACMI.
James E. Montie, MD is a consultant for Wilex AG.
Harris M. Nagler, MD is on the advisory committee for Boerhinger Ingelheim.
Glenn M. Preminger, MD is a consultant for Mission Pharmacal, Microvasive Urology, and Olympus Surgical America.
Bruce Shingleton, MD is on the speaker's bureau for Oncura.
Richard D. Williams, MD is an independent contractor and consultant and is on the speaker's bureau for Gyrus ACMI; and is on the speaker's bureau for AstraZeneca.

Disclosure of Discussion of non-FDA approved uses for pharmaceutical products and/or medical devices:
The University of Virginia School of Medicine, as an ACCME provider, requires that all faculty presenters identify and disclose any "off label" uses for pharmaceutical and medical device products. The University of Virginia School of Medicine recommends that each physician fully review all the available data on new products or procedures prior to instituting them with patients.

TO ENROLL

To enroll in the *Urologic Clinics of North America* Continuing Medical Education program, call customer service at 1-800-654-2452 or visit us online at www.theclinics.com/home/cme. The CME program is available to subscribers for an additional fee of $195.00

FORTHCOMING ISSUES

RECENT ISSUES

THE CLINICS ARE NOW AVAILABLE ONLINE!

Access your subscription at:
http://www.theclinics.com

UROLOGIC
CLINICS
of North America

Urol Clin N Am 33 (2006) xi–xii

Foreword

Urologic Imaging

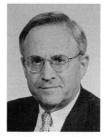

Martin I. Resnick, MD
Consulting Editor

The practice of urology has seen many innovations over the years and although we often are oriented toward those related to technological developments that impact our activities in the operating room, it is also important to recognize that technological changes have also had a significant impact on diagnostic urology as well. In the mid-1970s standard imaging included intravenous urography and when further evaluation of the urinary tract was required, additional studies typically included nephrotomography and renal angiography. Retrograde ureteropyelography was also commonly used because of the inability of these prior studies to consistently image the renal pelvis and ureter.

Clinical ultrasound developed in the 1970s and early A-mode instrumentation only allowed for delineation of interfaces, which was used for the assessment and aspiration of renal cysts. B-mode, gray scale, and improved resolution followed in addition to the development of color flow and power Doppler studies. Applications increased; renal masses were better defined and we are all familiar with the value of prostatic ultrasonography and how it has affected our specialty. CT scans further enhanced our ability to assess the urinary tract and not only were these studies of value for diagnostic purposes but they, in addition to ultrasound, allowed for the carrying out of biopsies, placement of percutaneous nephrostomies, and assessment of abnormalities in the kidney that previously had required surgical exploration. Magnetic resonance imaging and more recently positron emission tomography (PET) and single-photon emission computed tomography (SPECT) imaging have been used not only allowing for visualization of the urinary tract but also for better assessment of patients with malignancies to determine the extent of disease.

The current issue of *Urologic Clinics*, ably edited by Dr Pat Fulgham, clearly reviews many of these modalities. The monograph also uses the application of these imaging techniques in various areas including oncology, urologic trauma, and renal calculi. Updates are provided of these new modalities and their practical application is emphasized not only as used by radiologists but also how they may be applied to urologic practice.

Those who have been in practice for more than two decades can only be in awe of the many changes they have witnessed during their tenure as practicing urologists. We have gone from 2-dimensional static imaging to 3-dimensional imaging that allows not only for assessment of organ anatomy but of function as well. Urologists have benefited from these developments by improving the practice of our specialty but the true recipients are the patients who are better evaluated and subsequently treated.

Martin I. Resnick, MD
Department of Urology
Case Western Reserve University
School of Medicine/University Hospitals
11100 Euclid Avenue
Cleveland, OH 44106, USA

Preface

Urologic Imaging

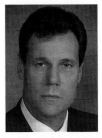

Pat Fox Fulgham, MD
Guest Editor

Imaging has always been a critical component of the practice of urology. Inherent in the procedure-oriented practice of urology is the need for imaging, both anatomical and functional. Since the days of cystoscopy by incandescent bulb, urologists have struggled to "see" the internal anatomy of patients. In perhaps no other specialty has imaging been so intimately bound up with diagnosis. The emergence of endoscopic, laparoscopic, and other minimally invasive procedures has been accompanied by an increasing dependence on imaging for their execution. The management of patients with urologic malignancies has placed imaging at the core of office practice. In all these areas, ie, diagnosis, treatment, and follow-up, we are blessed with almost daily innovations in imaging technology.

The nature of many urologic procedures requires that the clinician be able to perform imaging studies themselves. Urologists have therefore become adept at fluoroscopy and ultrasound sometimes without the benefit of formal training in their underlying physical principles. Tissue ablative procedures have made the extension of this expertise to CT and MRI scanning necessary.

Remote and robotic surgeries demand a familiarity with complex image manipulation. Urologists have realized that it is no longer sufficient to be able to interpret imaging studies but that they must also be able to perform them. With the performance of imaging studies comes the responsibility to thoroughly understand and to judiciously deploy the technology with quality control and patient safety as the guiding principles.

The trend in urologist-performed imaging studies, which began in conjunction with procedures, has recently been extended to the office environment. Increasingly, urologists are acquiring the equipment necessary to perform diagnostic and follow-up studies. There is an overwhelming economic and ethical need to behave responsibly by developing evidence-based indications for imaging. To develop such guidelines, urologists and others must understand the technical limitations as well as the potential benefits of each study.

The authors of the work presented in this issue have addressed imaging from the perspective of providing insight into the indications for studies based on the capabilities of each one. When

doi:10.1016/j.ucl.2006.04.001

appropriate, the technical aspects of the imaging modalities have been explained. Their excellent efforts should make it easier for all of us to use imaging in a safe and beneficial way.

Acknowledgments

I express my gratitude to Angela Clark for her expert assistance in editing and assembling this issue. Thanks to Catherine Bewick at Elsevier for her help and support.

Pat Fox Fulgham, MD
Urology Clinics of North Texas
8230 Walnut Hill Lane, Suite 700
Dallas, TX 75231, USA

E-mail address: pfulgham@airmail.net

ELSEVIER
SAUNDERS

Urol Clin N Am 33 (2006) 279–286

UROLOGIC
CLINICS
of North America

What's New in Urologic Ultrasound?

Eric A. Singer, MD, MA, Dragan J. Golijanin, MD,
Robert S. Davis, MD, Vikram Dogra, MD*

University of Rochester Medical Center, 601 Elmwood Avenue, Box 648, Rochester, NY 14642, USA

Ultrasonography allows providers to noninvasively image an area of interest in real time without the risks of ionizing radiation or nephrotoxic contrast agents. This article presents basic concepts of ultrasound along with new advances in ultrasound technology and their applications in small parts evaluation.

Ultrasound remains a key instrument in the diagnostic armamentarium of urologists. Ultrasonography allows providers to noninvasively image an area of interest in real time without the risks of ionizing radiation or nephrotoxic contrast agents. Since its first clinical applications in the 1940s, steady advances in ultrasound technology have continued to expand its role in the diagnosis, management, and follow-up of patients with urologic disorders [1]. This article presents basic concepts of ultrasound along with new advances in ultrasound technology and their applications in small parts evaluation.

Ultrasound physics

Ultrasound is based on the interpretation of sound waves that have been reflected by the interface of different tissues in the body. The fundamental principles of ultrasound include the piezoelectric effect, pulse–echo principle, and acoustic impedance.

The piezoelectric effect explains how mechanical energy and electrical energy are interconverted [2]. When pressure is applied to a quartz crystal, an electrical charge is created that is proportional to the force applied. Changing the polarity of a voltage applied to the transducer changes the thickness of the crystal, which expands and contracts as the polarity changes. This results in the generation of ultrasound waves that can be transmitted into the body. The emitted sound waves enter the body, and the vibrations of the reflected echoes are converted from mechanical energy to an electrical signal that is displayed as an image [3]. The pulse–echo principle states that the electrical impulse generated by reflected sound waves is proportional to the strength of the returning echo [3]. Acoustic impedance is a tissue-specific characteristic that is calculated by multiplying the density of the tissue scanned by the speed of the sound wave traveling through it. The degree to which ultrasound waves are reflected back to the probe is proportional to the density differences encountered between varying tissues, which are known as acoustic interfaces [3]. The density difference between air and tissue is so large that nearly all sound waves will be reflected back toward the transducer. Therefore a coupling medium, like ultrasound gel, is used to decrease the acoustic impedance between the transducer and skin to facilitate transmission of ultrasound waves.

When an area of interest is scanned by the ultrasound probe, most of the energy imparted is attenuated by absorption, reflection, and scattering, leaving little to be reflected back to the probe to form an image [4]. The degree of attenuation, or weakening of the sound wave's amplitude or intensity as it travels through tissue, is proportional to the frequency of the sound wave and proportional to the distance it has traversed. Shorter wavelengths (higher frequencies) are absorbed more rapidly by tissue and therefore have less

---

* Corresponding author.

E-mail address: vikram_dogra@urmc.rochester.edu (V. Dogra).

penetration. Higher frequencies, however, provide greater axial and lateral resolution. Frequency of the transducer has a direct relationship to resolution of the image and inverse relation to depth of penetration. Therefore, whenever possible, transducers of the highest permissible frequency should be used for scanning depending upon the depth of penetration required. Evaluation of the testes and penis ideally should be performed with a 10 to 14 MHz linear transducer.

Types of ultrasound

Two-dimensional ultrasound

Two-dimensional ultrasound is the technique most familiar to practicing urologists. All the currently used clinical ultrasound machines use B mode (brightness mode), where the reflected echoes appear as bright spots on the readout, with signal intensity being proportional to the brightness [5] (Fig. 1).

Color flow Doppler ultrasound

The Doppler effect is the change in frequency or wavelength of transmitted sound waves that occurs when there is relative motion between the transducer (sound source) and reflecting surfaces (red blood cells). This shift in frequency between the received and transmitted frequencies is measured in Hertz (Hz). This change can be represented either visually by color or by an audible signal. Pulsed duplex Doppler ultrasound allows for flow to be superimposed on the image as a continuous time–velocity waveform [4]. Color flow Doppler is extremely useful for evaluating testicular torsion and erectile dysfunction. Absence of color flow Doppler in the testis with high clinical index of suspicion is virtually diagnostic of

testicular torsion [6,7] (Fig. 2). Power Doppler ultrasound presents two-dimensional Doppler information by color-encoding the strength of the Doppler shifts. Power Doppler ultrasound is more sensitive in depicting slow flow in smaller and deeper vessels than color flow Doppler. Power Doppler scanning is valuable in scrotal ultrasonography because of its increased sensitivity to low-flow states and its independence from Doppler angle correction [6,7] (Fig. 2). Power Doppler ultrasound enhances the sensitivity of detecting blood flow by at least five times as compared with color flow Doppler ultrasound, but it does not provide a flow vector (direction of blood flow) or velocity [8,9].

Three-dimensional ultrasound

Three-dimensional ultrasound reconstructions are an exciting new development. They allow the creation of a three-dimensional image from a single sweep of the ultrasound probe that provides 360° viewing of the area scanned. This eliminates the problem of user-dependent variation in scanning, which is a significant problem with conventional two-dimensional ultrasound techniques [10]. Three-dimensional scanning also provides increased measuring accuracy, especially when looking at volumes, and allows for a better appreciation of the anatomic relationships between the

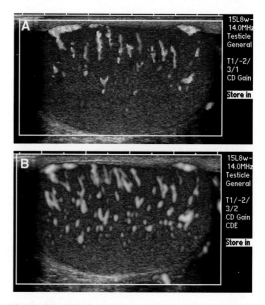

Fig. 2. (*A*) High-frequency transducer color flow Doppler of normal testis. (*B*) Demonstrates power Doppler appearance in a normal testis.

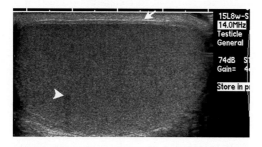

Fig. 1. Longitudinal sonogram of testis performed with high-frequency linear transducer demonstrates normal medium level echoes (arrow–tunica albuginea and arrowhead–vessel).

area of interest and its surrounding structures [4,10,11] (Fig. 3). Three-dimensional volume acquisition allows reconstruction of image in any plane, including coronal, sagittal, or axial planes (Fig. 4). Given these traits, three-dimensional ultrasounds allow much easier exam-to-exam comparison, making long-term follow-up possible without repeated exposures to radiation or nephrotoxic contrast agents [10,11]. In the adult population, three-dimensional studies of the prostate can provide more accurate calculations of PSA density and better treatment mapping for brachytherapy [10] (Fig. 5). Three-dimensional ultrasound may be used for routine evaluation of the testis. The main advantage of this technique is short image acquisition time, greater confidence in interpretation, and an ability to manipulate the image in any plane. This technique is also very useful for evaluating patients who have erectile dysfunction (Fig. 6).

Limitations in this technique include the requirement for highly trained technologists who are skilled in obtaining and manipulating the large data sets used in three-dimensional reconstruction. Artifacts can be introduced into the image during the initial scan or while it is being analyzed, resulting in possible misdiagnosis. Centers using three-dimensional ultrasound must invest in a computational infrastructure that can meet the hardware, software, storage, transfer/retrieval, and support requirements of this technology.

Four-dimensional ultrasound

Four-dimensional ultrasound incorporates a temporal dimension to three-dimensional ultrasound.

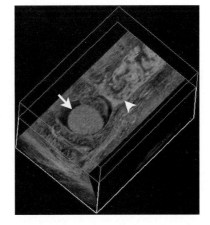

Fig. 4. Three-dimensional volume acquisition reveals testis (*arrow*) and spermatic cord (*arrowhead*) in a coronal plane. (*Courtesy of* GE Healthcare Technologies; with permission.)

This approach is useful for performing volume assessments as a function of time in dynamic systems, such as the cardiac cycle [12,13]. Four-dimensional ultrasound imaging also has been applied to interventional procedures such as solid organ biopsy [14]. Won and colleagues reported that four-dimensional ultrasound is a more intuitive modality for performing biopsies, because familiar two-dimensional images can be displayed for the operator while the volumetric processing is being performed. Additionally, presentation of four-dimensional reconstructions is continuous, thereby preventing time delays experienced with three-dimensional imaging [14]. As one would expect, the limitations of this technology are similar to those found with three-dimensional

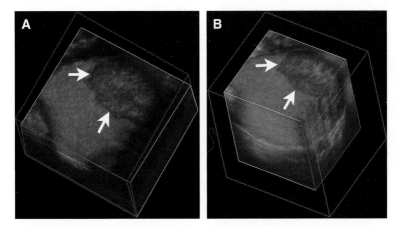

Fig. 3. (*A, B*) Three-dimensional volume acquisition of testis demonstrates a testicular mass (*arrows*) with well-defined relationship with its surrounding testicular parenchyma. (*Courtesy of* GE Healthcare Technologies; with permission.)

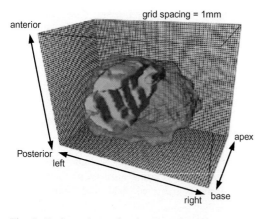

Fig. 5. Fusion volume showing B-mode surface (transparent) with reconstructed tumor (solid). The image was obtained using a GE Logiq700 US scanner and an electromagnetic positioning sensor from Ascension Technologies. (*Courtesy of* Benjamin Castaneda, Rochester, New York.)

imaging, namely the added bulk of the equipment and the technological sophistication.

Harmonic imaging ultrasound

Harmonic imaging is an ultrasound method in which the higher harmonic echoes (usually the second harmonic) of the fundamental (first harmonic) transmitted frequency are selectively detected and used for imaging. The higher harmonics may have been created by non-linear propagation of the ultrasound pulse. When

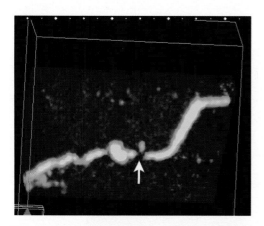

Fig. 6. Three-dimensional power Doppler sonogram with maximum intensity projection algorithm shows tortuous cavernosal artery caused by atherosclerosis with severe segmental stenosis (*arrow*) in a patient with erectile dysfunction.

harmonic B-mode imaging is used to improve image quality and contrast resolution of tissues, the technique is called tissue harmonic imaging. One of the main advantages of harmonic imaging is improved signal to noise ratio. Signal to noise ratio is the ratio of the amplitude of the desired signal (echoes forming the image) to the amplitude of noise signals (electronic noise not contributing to the image formation) at a given point in time. Other advantages include improved near field resolution (closer to the transducer) and improved contrast resolution (the ability to observe subtle changes between adjacent tissues). Pulse inversion harmonic imaging is used with ultrasound contrast agents (enhances image contrast) where identical ultrasonic pulses with opposite polarities are sent through an area of interest. Because the polarities are reversed, the linear aspects of the return signals cancel each other out, leaving only the nonlinear components (harmonic and subharmonic ultrasound waves) to form the image [15]. This technique enhances the nonlinear echoes formed by pulse inversion and is useful for examining low flow states [8].

Compound imaging

An array transducer is used to image the tissue of interest repeatedly by generating parallel sound waves aimed in offset directions [4]. The multiple return echoes then are averaged, and a single compound image is generated. This compounding can be achieved with frequency and temporal change. The advantage to this approach is that because multiple echoes are used to make the composite image, there is less graininess, speckle, and shadowing compared with conventional B mode imaging. There is a greater computational time with compound imaging and therefore a slower frame rate; however, the image has a higher contrast resolution and decreased artifacts such as side lobes (Fig. 7).

Extended field of view

Numerous images are obtained as the transducer is swept over the area of interest and the computer algorithm stores and analyzes the data. The acquired images then are overlapped appropriately to form an ultrasound image with a much larger field of view than what is possible with real-time imaging [4]. This mode is very useful when the testis is markedly enlarged and cannot fit in one view (Fig. 8).

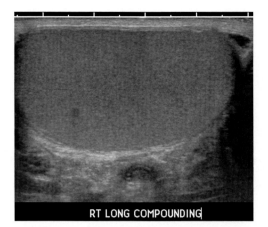

Fig. 7. Gray-scale two-dimensional imaging of right testis with compound image function demonstrates better resolution of the testicular parenchyma as compared with noncompound imaging as shown in Fig. 1.

Contrast agents in ultrasound

Contrast ultrasonography was applied first to imaging of the heart and liver, but it now is finding a greater role in evaluating the urology patient. The contrast agents used consist of intravenously injected microbubbles, which significantly increase the amount of ultrasonic reflection in the area of interest [16]. The ideal contrast agent must pass numerous hurdles. It should have the ability to survive its journey through the circulatory system, be easily administered without significant adverse effects or allergic potential, and be safe to use in patients with marginal renal function (ie, not be nephrotoxic) [16].

The most important phenomena involved in ultrasound–contrast agent interactions involve the scattering. Scattering of ultrasound occurs when an ultrasound wave is traveling through a medium that contains localized inhomogeneities such as small particles or bubbles. Laboratory study and clinical observations have demonstrated that ultrasound contrast agents are very efficacious scatterers of ultrasound, capable of producing much stronger backscatter than regular blood or normal tissue, because of the extremely large difference between the acoustic impedances of the gas inside the bubbles and the surrounding liquid. Such bubbles react to the external ultrasound pressure field with volume pulsations, absorbing and radiating ultrasound energy, thus generating a scattered field and reducing the transmitted field. Scattering is especially pronounced at the resonant frequency of a contrast agent. For an air-filled bubble in water, this frequency (in megahertz) is approximately equal to 3/R, where R is the bubble radius in micrometers. For example, the resonant frequency for a 1 μm bubble will be 3 MHz, which is close to the frequency range used in diagnostic ultrasound [8].

Contrast ultrasound is used with harmonic imaging techniques that rely on the nonlinear behavior pattern of the microbubble contrast [16,17]. When microbubbles are exposed to enough sonic energy from the ultrasound probe, they display nonlinear behavior, because they are able to expand more than they can contract. Nonlinear interaction phenomena include harmonic and subharmonic generation. The spectrum of the scattered ultrasound signal will contain higher harmonics of the incident or fundamental frequency in addition to the original incident frequency. Highly nonlinear systems, contrast agent bubbles can generate subharmonic backscatter at a frequency equal to half of the incident frequency [8,18].

The indications for contrast ultrasonography often overlap with those for contrast CT. Robbin and colleagues indicated that this technology has the potential for evaluating renal masses by using noncontrast ultrasound followed by contrast ultrasound scans, looking for enhancement of hypervascular lesions secondary to the increased number of microbubbles present in the mass [16]. They also proposed a contrast ultrasound-specific classification pattern for complicated renal cysts. This pattern is a modification of the Bosniak criteria used in CT [16]. Additional work with this technology is ongoing and focuses on using contrast ultrasound for assessing renal perfusion, infarction, pyelonephritis, and intraoperatively for localizing tumors [16].

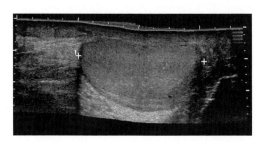

Fig. 8. Gray-scale sonogram of left testis with extended field of view.

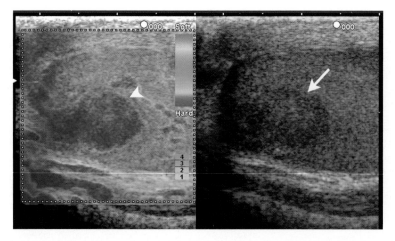

Fig. 9. Gray scale image of the testis reveals an intratesticular well-circumscribed hypoechoic mass (*arrow*), seen as a dark blue area (*arrowhead*) on corresponding sonoelastogram. Note blue color represents hard area. This was proven to be a seminoma. (*Courtesy of* Leo Pellwein, MD, Innsbruck Austria.)

Sonoelastography

This imaging approach attempts to provide a real-time visual depiction of the visco–elastic properties of tissue that typically are assessed by means of manual palpation [19]. By using the principle of sonoelastography to increase the sensitivity and objectivity of a traditional physical examination, it may be possible to detect tumors earlier in their course because of their increased hardness as compared with the surrounding tissue. Once it is a proven technology, genitourinary sonoelastography can be applied readily to the evaluation of the prostate and testicles (Fig. 9)

Compact ultrasound systems

Owing to advances in technology in the field of ultrasound and computers, ultrasound systems have progressed from room size equipment to small handheld devices. The size and weight of ultrasound systems have continued to decrease, and so have the production costs. The image resolution and its features continue to improve. With affordable prices and better image resolution, these compact systems have become more attractive to medical specialists, prompting them to use imaging devices as a part of their routine practice [4,20]. The American Institute of Ultrasound in Medicine has brought together a multi-disciplinary panel of experts to address the opportunities and challenges inherent in the dissemination of ultrasound technology [20].

They concluded that all practitioners who use ultrasound be appropriately trained in its use and committed to ongoing education, professional development, and outcomes-based research to ensure optimal patient care.

Animal imaging in genitourinary ultrasound

High-resolution animal research ultrasound machines are available for genitourinary research with two- and three-dimensional capability. These ultrasound machines use extremely high frequency transducers of 40 MHz (Fig. 10).

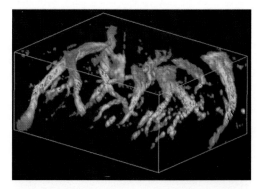

Fig. 10. Three-dimensional power Doppler of adult mouse testicle. Static image using three-dimensional power Doppler of perfusion in adult mouse testicle. The image of the testicle was constructed with multiple two-dimensional slices to create the three-dimensional volumetric image. (*Courtesy of* VisualSonics, Inc., Toronto, ON; with permission.)

Table 1
Innovations in ultrasound and the resulting improvement in imaging

Innovation	Result
Improved ergonomics	Decreased work related injuries
Image resolution	Enhanced definition of tissue interfaces
Compact size	Portable, bedside imaging
Three-and four-dimensional	View area of interest from any angle
Harmonic imaging	Better tissue definition; often used with contrast agents
Compound imaging	Decreased graininess/ speckle/shadowing
Extended field of view	View a larger area of interest
Contrast agents	Assess vascularity or enhancement without nephrotoxicity
Sonoelastography	Earlier detection of tumor

Forthcoming advances

Capacitative micromachined ultrasonic transducers

Capacitative micromachined ultrasonic transducers are transducers constructed of new materials such as silicon wafers rather than piezoelectric crystals [21]. The hope is that this technology will allow one single transducer head to have the functionality to generate multiple frequencies and wavelengths, eliminating the need to use several transducers during an examination.

Summary

Ultrasound technology and its application to urologic disease continue to advance. Conventional two-dimensional ultrasound remains an integral piece of the practicing urologist's diagnostic armamentarium. Contrast agents allow for the assessment of vascularity and flow states previously possible only with CT and MRI. Multi-dimensional imaging provides powerful and detailed spatial relationships that can be reviewed from any angle and readily compared over time. Urologists must continue to familiarize themselves with these new aspects of ultrasonography and work collaboratively with their counterparts in radiology to ensure that the highest standards of care are provided to patients. New advances in ultrasound technology are summarized in Table 1.

References

[1] Resnick MI. Ultrasonography of the prostate and testes. J Ultrasound Med 2003;22:869–77.

[2] Rozycki GS. Surgeon-performed ultrasound: its use in clinical practice. Ann Surg 1998;228:16–28.

[3] McAchran SE, Dogram V, Resnick MI. Office urologic ultrasound. Urol Clin North Am 2005;32: 337–52.

[4] Hangiandreou NJ. AAPM/RSNA physics tutorial for residents. Topics in US. B-mode US: basics concepts and new technology. Radiographics 2003;23: 1019–33.

[5] Resnick MI. Ultrasonography. In: Resnick MI, Novick AC, editors. Urology secrets. Philadelphia: Hanley & Belfus; 1999. p. 14.

[6] Dogra V, Bhatt S. Acute painful scrotum. Radiol Clin North Am 2004;42:349–63.

[7] Dogra VS, Gottlieb RH, Oka M, et al. Sonography of the scrotum. Radiology 2003;227:18–36.

[8] Dogra V, Rubens D, editors. Ultrasound secrets. Philadelphia: Hanley & Belfus; 2004.

[9] Hamper UM, DeJong MR, Caskey CI, et al. Power Doppler imaging: clinical experience and correlation with color Doppler US and other imaging modalities. Radiographics 1997;17:499–513.

[10] Downey DB, Fenster A, Williams JC. Clinical utility of three-dimensional US. Radiographics 2000;20: 559–71.

[11] Riccabona M, Fritz GA, Schollnast H, et al. Hydronephrotic kidney: pediatric three-dimensional US for relative renal size assessment— initial experience. Radiology 2005;236(1):276–83.

[12] Bhat AH, Corbett VN, Liu R, Carpenter ND, et al. Validation of volume and mass assessments for human fetal heart imaging by four-dimensional spatiotemporal image correlation echocardiography. J Ultrasound Med 2004;23:1151–9.

[13] Nguyen LD, Leger C, Debrun D, et al. Validation of a volumic reconstruction in 4-d echocardiography and gated spect using a dynamic cardiac phantom. Ultrasound Med Biol 2003;29(8):1151–60.

[14] Won HJ, Han JK, Do KH, et al. Values of four-dimensional ultrasonography in ultrasonographically guided biopsies of hepatic masses. J Ultrasound Med 2003;22:215–20.

[15] Kim TK, Choi BI, Han JK, et al. Hepatic tumors: contrast agent-enhancement patterns with pulse-inversion harmonic US. Radiology 2000;216: 411–7.

[16] Robbin ML, Lockhart ME, Barr RG. Renal imaging with ultrasound contrast: current status. Radiol Clin N Am 2003;41:963–78.

[17] Burns PN. Harmonic imaging with ultrasound contrast agents. Clin Radiol 1996;51(Suppl 1): 50–5.

[18] Goldberg BB, Liu JB, Forsberg F. Ultrasound contrast agents: a review. Ultrasound Med Biol 1994;20: 319–33.

[19] Hall TJ. AAPM/RSNA physics tutorial for residents: topics in US. Beyond the basics: elasticity imaging with US. Radiographics 2003;23:1657–71.

[20] Greenbaum LD, Benson CB, Nelson LH, et al. Proceedings of the compact ultrasound conference sponsored by the American Institute of Ultrasound in Medicine. J Ultrasound Med 2004; 23:1249–54.

[21] Ergun AS, Huang Y, Zhuang X, et al. Capacitative micromachined ultrasonic transducers: fabrication technology. IEEE Trans Ultrason Ferroelectr Freq Control 2005;52:2242–58.

ELSEVIER
SAUNDERS

Urol Clin N Am 33 (2006) 287–300

UROLOGIC
CLINICS
of North America

Maximizing Clinical Information Obtained by CT

Fadi N. Joudi, MD[a,*], David M. Kuehn, MD[b],
Richard D. Williams, MD[a]

[a]Department of Urology, University of Iowa, 200 Hawkins Drive, 3 RCP, Iowa City, IA 52242, USA
[b]Department of Radiology, University of Iowa, 200 Hawkins Drive, 3 JPP, Iowa City, IA 52242, USA

Radiologic imaging, especially CT scanning, constitutes an integral part of any urologist's practice. Advances in the past decade in using CT scan to diagnose nephrolithiasis, along with progress in developing multidetector CT (MDCT) and 3D reconstruction, have revolutionized the value of CT in urology. In many institutions, CT has replaced intravenous (IV) pyelograms. CT scans performed dynamically through the unenhanced, nephrographic, and excretory phases may replace other imaging tests to evaluate hematuria. Staging of urologic malignancies includes a CT scan of the abdomen. Preoperative planning for living related kidney donors using CT angiograms has become common practice in transplant centers. Additionally, the widespread use of CT in evaluating abdominal pain has led to an increase in diagnosis of incidental urologic findings. This article describes recent developments in CT and its use in urologic practice, and how the urologist can maximize clinical information obtained by it.

Basics of CT imaging

Principles

As with conventional radiographic images, the basis for CT images is the attenuation of x-ray photons as they pass through the patient. In CT, a computer mathematically reconstructs a cross-sectional image of the body from measurements of x-ray transmission through thin slices of body tissue [1]. A thin, collimated x-ray beam is generated on one side of the patient and the amount of transmitted radiation is measured by detectors on the opposite side. These measurements are repeated systematically many times while a series of exposures from different projections is made as the x-ray beam rotates about the patient.

Practical points about contrast media and toxicity

Commonly, oral contrast agents are administered before scanning for bowel opacification to help differentiate bowel from tumors, lymph nodes, abscesses, and hematomas. Oral contrast is less critical in urologic imaging than in gastrointestinal imaging; and in certain situations, such as evaluation for renal calculi or CT angiography, the use of oral contrast may be counterproductive [2].

IV contrast aids in the depiction of small lesions by increasing their conspicuity, in the demonstration of vascular anatomy and vessel patency, and in the characterization of lesions through their patterns of contrast enhancement. The commercially available radiographic contrast agents are tri-iodinated derivatives of benzoic acid. All the currently available IV contrast media are excreted by way of the kidney through glomerular filtration, with no significant tubular excretion or resorption [3].

It is prudent that the physician inquire about the patient's history, including renal function and history of previous allergies to contrast material. A history of asthma and severe allergies increases the risk of subsequent reaction to contrast agent injection by a small percentage [4]. Allergy to

* Corresponding author.
   E-mail address: fadi-joudi@uiowa.edu (F.N. Joudi).

shellfish is not associated with increased risk of re-action to contrast [5]. The use of corticosteroids with or without antihistamines 12 hours before contrast injection to reduce the occurrence of ad-verse reactions in allergic patients has been well established [6].

Contrast nephropathy (CN) is defined as an acute impairment of renal function after expo-sure to a radiographic contrast medium. It is typically reversible, although cases of permanent nephrotoxicity, especially when the renal failure is oliguric, have been reported [7]. The most im-portant risk factor for development of CN is pre-existing renal insufficiency [7]. The presence of diabetes is not an independent risk factor, but is a major contributing factor in the presence of renal insufficiency. Other risk factors include dehydration, poor renal perfusion as in conges-tive heart failure, and the presence of other fac-tors that may be nephrotoxic, such as certain medications [5]. The first step to prevent CN is adequate hydration, either orally or intrave-nously [8]. Avoiding multiple imaging studies with contrast injection within a short period of time and using alternate noncontrast studies that can answer the diagnostic question can be helpful as well. N-acetylcysteine has been advo-cated as a protective agent, being a vasodilator and free radical scavenger [9]. Iodixanol, the only available nonionic, iso-osmolar, iodinated contrast agent, was shown to have a protective effect in two small studies [10,11]. There is evi-dence of a slightly higher incidence of CN when high-osmolality versus low-osmolality con-trast agents are used [7].

The urologist and radiologist should be aware of patients who have diabetes and are taking metformin [4]. Metformin is excreted by the kidney unchanged and patients who have re-nal insufficiency will have higher than expected serum levels of metformin, putting them at risk for lactic acidosis [12]. Because IV contrast agents can lead to acute alteration in renal func-tion, the US Food and Drug Administration currently recommends that metformin be with-held for 48 hours at the time an iodinated IV contrast agent is administered, and reinstituted only after renal function has been re-evaluated and found to be normal.

Phases of CT imaging

Multiphase enhanced CT scans tend to char-acterize renal masses better than single-phase enhanced imaging [13]. A comprehensive CT scan of the urinary tract includes

- An unenhanced axial CT scan of the kidneys
- An enhanced CT scan of the abdomen and pelvis
- Excretory phase enhanced images of the uri-nary tract obtained with axial CT images

Unenhanced CT images are used to evaluate for stone disease and renal parenchymal calcifica-tions; for precontrast attenuation measurements of renal masses; and to assist in excluding hemorrhagic changes [14]. Some investigators include arterial phase images at 25 seconds to evaluate for vascular abnormalities, such as arte-riovenous malformations, and to demonstrate the vascular anatomy in surgical candidates [15]. Nephrographic phase images obtained at 90 to 180 seconds are useful in the evaluation of renal parenchyma for neoplasms, scarring, and inflam-matory disease. Some investigators advocate the addition of a corticomedullary phase at 30 to 70 seconds to characterize renal masses better and particularly to evaluate the liver better [16]. The renal veins can be evaluated for possible tumor in-vasion during the nephrographic phase. Delayed images are obtained after contrast is excreted into the collecting system and are usually obtained at 3 to 5 minutes. These images may be useful in evaluating central renal masses and urothelial ab-normalities. The bladder is seen best in 20-minute and postvoid images.

Hounsfield units

CT creates an image of the body from mea-surements of linear attenuation collected from multiple projections around a thin tomographic slice [3]. A cross-sectional view of a layer of the body is divided into many tiny blocks (pixels) from which a reconstructed image is displayed. The gray scale of each pixel on CT is a function of the amount of radiation absorbed at that point, which is termed an attenuation value, expressed in Hounsfield units (HU). The attenuation value as-signed to each pixel is based on a reference scale in which −1000 HU is the value assigned to air, +1000 HU to dense bone, and 0 HU to water. User selection of the number of shades of gray (window width) in the image and the central hue of gray (window level) permits modification of im-age contrast. By adjusting the window width and level, the image can be optimized for evaluating very dense structures such as bone and the contrast-filled bladder, very light structures such as the lung, and very subtle structures such as a solid tumor within normal parenchyma.

Multidetector or Multichannel CT

The single-slice spiral CT, introduced for clinical use in 1988 [17], has now evolved into MDCT. In MDCT there are multiple rows of detectors (currently up to 64) instead of a single row [18]. Thus, MDCT allows multiple channels of data to be acquired simultaneously, permitting thinly collimated images to be obtained through the entire abdomen in a single breath hold. The advantages of MDCT include

- Improved temporal resolution (faster scanning results in fewer motion artifacts)
- Improved spatial resolution (thinner sections improve resolution in the z axis (along the table), reducing partial-volume artifacts and increasing diagnostic accuracy)
- Increased concentration of intravascular contrast material (because scanning is done more quickly, contrast material can be administered at a faster rate, improving the conspicuity of arteries and veins)
- Efficient x-ray tube use (a shorter scanning time leads to diminished x-ray tube heating, thus shortening the delay for x-ray tube cooling between scans, which is critical in multiphase examinations)
- Longer anatomic coverage (the multiple detectors allow scanning of a larger anatomic area because of the simultaneous registration of multiple sections during each rotation and the increased gantry rotation speed)

MDCT offers greater speed of acquisition and higher resolution images than single-detector CT, allowing multiplanar imaging and making 3D reconstruction feasible. A 16-slice MDCT can acquire images of the chest, abdomen, and pelvis in 20 seconds. The application of 3D techniques to CT allows for accurate depiction of tumor depth and location and relationship of tumor to adjacent structures, and delineation of renal vascular anatomy [19]. The location of the kidney in relation to the rib cage, iliac crest, and spine can aid preoperative planning, especially in the setting of a nephron-sparing procedure [20]. Triphasic (unenhanced, enhanced early vascular, and delayed parenchymal phase) helical CT is performed with acquisition of datasets for subsequent 3D imaging using a volume-rendering workstation. One major application of 3D CT in urology is CT urography because it provides a complete evaluation of the collecting system [21].

CT applications in urology

Urolithiasis

Patients who have flank pain and are suspected of having renal colic have been evaluated traditionally using IV urography (IVU). Although the reported sensitivity of IVU is relatively high (84%–95%), it is associated with inherent limitations, such as lower sensitivity for small stones and stones with low radiation attenuation, the need for contrast agents, and the limitations of projection radiography [22]. Since the first report by Smith and colleagues [23] in 1995 on the use of unenhanced CT for identifying urolithiasis, CT has become the standard diagnostic technique for evaluating patients who have renal colic. The advantages of CT over IVU include a faster examination speed, avoidance of IV contrast, and the ability to diagnose alternative abdominal pathologies that mimic the symptoms of renal colic [24,25]. Unenhanced CT for stone detection has been reported to have sensitivities ranging from 96% to 100% and specificities ranging from 92% to 100% [22].

Almost all renal and ureteral stones are detected at helical CT because the attenuation of stones is inherently higher than that of the surrounding tissues [26]. One exception is the indinavir stone, which is seen in patients who have human immunodeficiency syndrome taking this protease inhibitor. The medication can crystallize in the urine and result in stones that may not be detected by CT [27].

The most common locations for obstruction by a stone include the natural anatomic points of narrowing: the ureteropelvic junction, the pelvic brim where the ureter crosses the iliac vessels, and the ureterovesical junction. The most obvious sign of a ureteral stone is an area of high attenuation within the ureter which appears similar in density to calcium on CT. At times, a stone can be difficult to differentiate from a phlebolith, making it necessary to look for secondary signs of obstruction, which include ureteral dilation, asymmetric inflammatory change of the perinephric fat, hydronephrosis, and nephromegaly [28,29]. The soft tissue "rim" sign, which refers to a soft tissue ring surrounding the calcification, represents the edematous ureteral wall and can be useful in differentiating a phlebolith from a ureteral stone (Fig. 1) [30]. Another helpful sign to differentiate a phlebolith is the comet sign; the calcified phlebolith represents the comet nucleus, and the adjacent, tapering, noncalcified portion of the vein is the comet tail [31]. An obstructing stone at the ureterovesical junction can be difficult to differentiate from a stone that recently passed into the bladder. In such a case, it may be helpful to place the patient in the prone position and obtain a repeat image of the pelvis. A stone that falls to the anterior portion of the bladder is a stone that has passed [32].

Hematuria work-up and CT urogram

The evaluation of hematuria is a common reason for a urology referral. Historically, the work-up included IVU, urine cytology, and cystoscopy. Other imaging modalities available for hematuria work-up include CT, ultrasonography, MRI, and retrograde pyelography. Occasionally, the urologist will need more than one modality to complete the work-up. With the advent of MDCT, it is possible to perform a comprehensive evaluation of a patient who has hematuria with a single examination [33]. The unenhanced phase of CT can help diagnose urolithiasis, the enhanced nephrographic phase aids in detection of renal parenchymal masses, and the excretory phase with 3D reformation allows evaluation of the entire urothelium (Fig. 2). Some investigators add a corticomedullary phase to characterize parenchymal renal masses better [34]. MDCT has been shown to have high sensitivity in detecting upper tract urothelial cancers [35]. One concern about this comprehensive CT technique is radiation dose to the patient, and some investigators advocate not

covering the entire abdomen and pelvis in all phases of the examination, to limit the radiation dose [36]. Other investigators have suggested obtaining a post-CT conventional radiograph that can substitute for the excretory phase of the CT [14] to provide images in a format more familiar to urologists; however, it may entail transferring the patient from the CT suite to the fluoroscopy suite. Patient transfer can be avoided if the CT room has a ceiling-mounted x-ray tube. Initial reports about conventional CT for detecting upper tract urothelial cancer have shown limitations in the sensitivity of this modality [37,38]. CT urography, however, has been reported to have high sensitivity in detecting urothelial lesions. In a group of 57 subjects who presented with hematuria, 38 subjects were found to have intrinsic urothelial lesions, of whom 15 had urothelial cancer [39]. CT urography allowed detection of 37 lesions with a sensitivity of 97%, whereas retrograde pyelography allowed detection of 31 lesions with a sensitivity of 82%. Caoili and colleagues [40] report that MDCT urography can detect most upper tract urothelial carcinomas. In their series of 18 subjects, 89% of malignant upper tract foci were detectable with MDCT urography. Although neither IVU nor CT is as sensitive as cystoscopy in detecting urothelial tumors in the bladder, large bladder tumors can be visualized with imaging studies because they appear as filling defects in the bladder lumen or as focal nodular bladder wall thickening [14].

Solid and cystic renal masses

CT is an excellent imaging modality for the evaluation of a renal mass. A renal mass can be characterized as a simple cyst, a complex cyst, or a solid mass. Solid masses that enhance by more

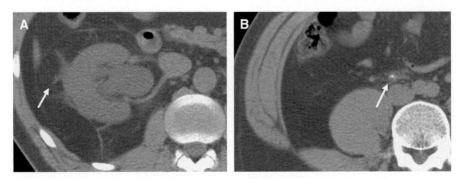

Fig. 1. Obstructing ureteral stone. (*A*) Hydronephrosis of the right kidney with perinephric stranding (*arrow*). (*B*) Dense ureteral stone with the soft tissue rim sign (*arrow*) and periureteral stranding.

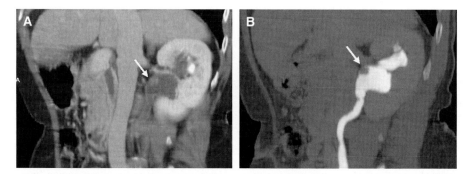

Fig. 2. Transitional cell carcinoma. (*A*) Coronal reconstruction in the venous phase showing a transitional cell carcinoma as an enhancing nodule (*arrow*) arising from the mucosa of the left renal pelvis. (*B*) Coronal reconstruction in the delayed or excretory phase showing the nodule as a filling defect (*arrow*).

than 20 HU are almost always malignant, with the exception of angiomyolipoma [41]. The presence of even a small amount of fat within a renal mass on CT scan, confirmed by an enhancement of less than 10 HU, virtually excludes the diagnosis of renal cell carcinoma and is considered diagnostic of angiomyolipoma (Fig. 3) [42]. Papillary renal cancers enhance less intensely than other cell types; these lesions accumulate contrast material more slowly, and delayed images may be helpful in confirming enhancement [43].

Renal masses are evaluated best using the multiphasic CT. Unenhanced images are performed to detect calcifications within the lesion and provide a baseline density to allow evaluation of enhancement. The nephrographic phase helps characterize the renal mass and detect any enhancement after IV contrast is injected; homogenous enhancement of the renal veins during this phase is also helpful to evaluate for renal venous invasion [2]. The excretory phase is useful in

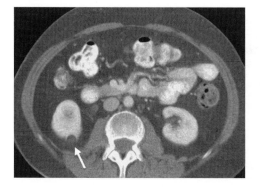

Fig. 3. Angiomyelolipoma appears as a fat density lesion in the posterior cortex of the right kidney (*arrow*).

assessing central renal masses, to help differentiate renal cell cancer from urothelial cancer.

If a solid mass is detected on contrast CT with no precontrast images to calculate enhancement, then delayed images 30 minutes to 4 hours later showing de-enhancement may be helpful [2]. Vascular masses, such as renal cancer, decrease in density on delayed images, and some investigators suggest a decrease of 15 HU or more is consistent with tumor [2]. A hyperdense cyst, on the other hand, shows no change in density between the postcontrast and the delayed phase images [44]. Some investigators have suggested obtaining portal venous phase images at 70 seconds to differentiate renal cell cancer from a hyperdense cyst, with attenuation greater than 70 HU favoring a diagnosis of renal cancer [45].

Renal cysts are a common radiologic finding and may present a management dilemma for the urologist. Ultrasound is a useful modality in evaluating renal cysts [46]. CT helps to characterize renal cysts by assessing wall thickness, presence and thickness of septa, calcifications, cyst attenuation (density), and foci of enhancement. Calcifications in a renal cystic mass have been investigated and found to be present in both benign and malignant lesions [47]; these calcifications are not as important as the presence of associated soft tissue elements. Often, cystic renal masses are characterized according to the Bosniak classification system [46–48]. A recent update of this classification system has been published by Israel and Bosniak [49].

The most important criterion used to differentiate surgical lesions from nonsurgical lesions is the presence or absence of tissue vascularity (enhancement). Categories I, II, and IIF lesions do not measurably enhance. Category I lesions are benign simple cysts with a hairline thin wall, which do not contain septa, calcifications, or solid components. It measures water density and does not enhance. Category II lesions are slightly more complicated and may contain thin calcifications, high attenuation fluid, and few thin septa in which "perceived" enhancement may be present. Perceived enhancement is seen when the thin smooth septa and walls of these lesions enhance subjectively when the unenhanced and contrast-enhanced images are compared side by side, and is believed to be caused by contrast material within the tiny capillaries in the wall and septa of these benign lesions. Uniformly high attenuation lesions of less than 3 cm (so-called high-density cysts) that are well marginated and do not enhance are included in this group. Category III lesions are more complex and may contain foci of calcification and irregular or smooth walls or septa in which measurable enhancement is present. Cystic masses that are difficult to categorize as II or III lesions are labeled as IIF, or cysts that warrant close follow-up. These include cysts that may contain multiple hairline thin septa or minimal smooth thickening of their wall or septa. Perceived enhancement of their septa or wall may be present. Their wall or septa may contain calcification that may be thick and nodular, but no measurable contrast enhancement is present. These lesions are generally well marginated. Totally intrarenal nonenhancing high-attenuation renal lesions of greater than 3 cm are also included in this category [47]. Category IV lesions are cystic masses that can have all the criteria of category III lesions, but also contain enhancing soft tissue components adjacent to, but independent of, the wall or septum (Fig. 4). Category I and II lesions

are considered benign, whereas category III and IV lesions are possibly malignant and necessitate further definition.

Preoperative evaluation for living renal donors

The advent of laparoscopic donor nephrectomy in 1995 has increased the number of available donors because of reduced postoperative pain and recovery time [50]. This procedure is associated with several technical challenges, including a limited surgical field of view. Consequently, a preoperative evaluation of the donor anatomy is critical. Information about the renal artery anatomy and the length and number of renal veins is required [51]. Traditionally, potential donors have been evaluated with IVU and renal angiography, but this has been replaced by CT angiography [52]. More recently, MDCT has been shown to be useful for angiographic applications because it provides more complete anatomic coverage, increased contrast enhancement of the arteries, greater longitudinal spatial resolution, and more detailed and sensitive depiction of the renal vessels (Fig. 5) [51,53].

Some investigators recommend precontrast CT imaging to rule out nephrolithiasis, because it would be an important finding in potential renal donors, whereas others omit that phase to decrease radiation dose [51,53]. Renal artery and venous anatomy are evaluated on arterial phase images; if the renal veins are not enhanced during the arterial phase, then venous phase images at 55 seconds are obtained [51]. Suspicious renal masses, a donor exclusion criterion, are detected best during the nephrographic phase. The collecting system is assessed either with a delayed topogram, a 3D reconstruction, or conventional

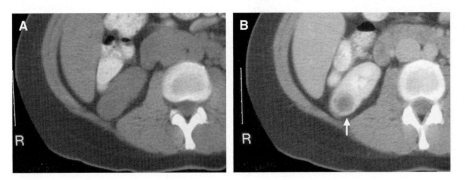

Fig. 4. Bosniak type III cyst in the lower pole of the right kidney. (*A*) Precontrast and (*B*) venous phase images showing a thick enhancing wall (*arrow*).

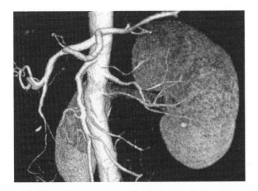

Fig. 5. Three left renal arteries demonstrated in a 3D reconstructed image of the kidney in a potential donor.

radiography using a lower radiation dose. Three-dimensional CT angiogram images can be obtained using either volume rendering or maximum intensity projection images, especially for the depiction of small vessels [51]. The end result is a format that is familiar to most surgeons for use in preoperative planning. An alternative imaging modality that can be used in patients allergic to IV contrast and that has been shown to be helpful for preoperative planning is 3D magnetic resonance angiography [54].

Ureteropelvic junction obstruction

Ureteropelvic junction obstruction generally implies a congenital proximal ureteric obstruction detected in utero or later in life, although the exact cause is unclear. Intrinsic abnormalities of collagen or muscle and crossing vessels are potential causes. Traditionally, this condition has been evaluated by IVU or retrograde pyelograms. However, these examinations only demonstrate the lumen of the ureter and do not allow direct visualization of extrinsic abnormalities such as a crossing vessel [36]. The increasing use of minimally invasive procedures such as endopyelotomy necessitates a precise anatomic evaluation of the ureteropelvic junction and any crossing vasculature [55]. Endoscopic repair of ureteropelvic junction obstruction can be performed using a blind incision in the posterior ureteral wall, and a potential complication occurs if the incision encounters an abnormally positioned renal vessel [2]. MDCT angiography and urography with 3D reconstructions can depict the collecting system, the ureters, and the vasculature in a format that is familiar to urologists and can help prevent such problems [36]. It can demonstrate the presence of crossing

vessels and indicate whether they correspond to the level of the focal ureteral obstruction [55]. The CT protocol involves arterial and venous phase contrast-enhanced images with approximately 30- and 60-second delays, respectively [55]. In addition to hydronephrosis, certain findings on CT often lead to the suggestion of ureteropelvic junction obstruction [55], including

- Rotation of the affected kidney in the axial plane with the hilum facing anteriorly, and in the coronal plane with the upper pole deviated laterally
- Lack of perinephric stranding, reflecting a chronic state
- Asymmetry of the rate and degree of corticomedullary and ureteropelvic opacification
- Presence of cortical thinning
- Hydronephrosis of the extrarenal collecting system more than the intrarenal portion, that assumes an inverted teardrop shape tapering to the point of transition

Three-dimensional CT angiography and urography have been shown to be of value in weighing or considering currently available treatment options, and may influence the selection of management options of retrograde endopyelotomy or surgical dismembered pyeloplasty (open or laparoscopic) [56,57].

Bladder abnormalities

Bladder conditions that can cause hematuria and voiding symptoms include neoplasms, stones, cystitis, and diverticula. Imaging modalities for evaluating the bladder include ultrasonography, CT, MRI, IVU, and cystography. Bladder distention is essential for optimal CT evaluation. The bladder is visualized with contrast excreted by the kidneys or directly instilled through a foley catheter [36]. Flat tumors or small papillary tumors of the bladder can be missed with CT, and cystoscopy remains the standard for evaluating the bladder for neoplasms.

Adrenal imaging

Incidental adrenal masses are found in 5% of patients undergoing abdominal CT [58]. Differential diagnosis of an adrenal mass includes adrenal adenoma, primary cortical carcinoma, myelolipoma, pheochromocytoma, and metastatic lesion. Most adrenal masses are adenomas, even in patients who have extra-adrenal malignancy [58]. In this group of patients, differentiating adenomas from metastases is important to determine the appropriate therapy. MRI is a very useful modality in defining adrenal masses [59]. Many studies have evaluated the usefulness of CT attenuation measurements at both unenhanced and delayed contrast-enhanced CT to differentiate benign from malignant lesions [60–66]. These studies have used two independent properties of adenomas that can be evaluated with CT to characterize these lesions. First, most adenomas contain large amounts of intracellular lipids, resulting in lower attenuation values than nonadenomas at unenhanced CT [67]. Second, all adenomas, including those without substantial lipid content, tend to have a more rapid loss of attenuation value soon after enhancement with contrast material. Many of these studies have attempted to detect threshold attenuation values to differentiate adenomas from nonadenomas. Boland and colleagues [61] performed a meta-analysis of 10 CT studies and concluded that a threshold of 10 HU or less on unenhanced CT corresponded to a sensitivity of 71% and specificity of 98% in the diagnosis of adrenal adenomas. For patients found to have an incidental adrenal adenoma that did not have an

unenhanced CT, some investigators have suggested using enhancement washout curves at 15-minute delayed images to distinguish adenomas from nonadenomas, to avoid the cost and inconvenience of having the patient return for a repeat CT scan. [66,68]. Caoili and colleagues [67] evaluated adrenal masses using both properties, with a protocol consisting of unenhanced CT. Enhanced and delayed enhanced CT images were obtained for those with attenuation values greater than 10 HU. An adenoma was diagnosed if a mass had an attenuation value of 10 HU or less at unenhanced CT, or a percentage enhancement washout value of 60% or higher (Fig. 6). Using this protocol, the investigators reported a sensitivity of 98% and specificity of 92% in detecting adrenal adenomas. Other investigators felt that this approach may not be practical because of the 15-minute window necessary to review and interpret the CT findings to determine whether there is a need for a repeat delayed scanning, while the patient is kept in the CT department [69].

Adrenal myelolipoma is an uncommon benign tumor composed of mature adipose cells and hematopoietic tissue, with characteristic CT

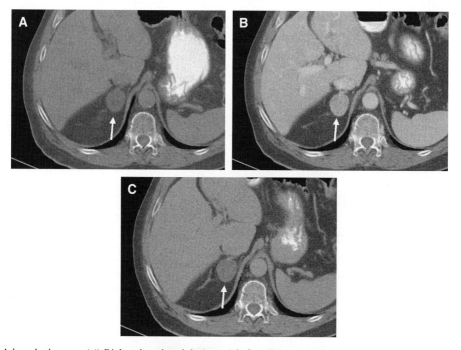

Fig. 6. Adrenal adenoma. (*A*) Right adrenal nodule (*arrow*) before IV contrast has a 6 HU density measurement. (*B*) Venous phase; nodule intensity measures 108 HU. (*C*) Delayed or washout phase; 31 HU. This finding is diagnostic of an adrenal adenoma by both CT attenuation criteria; it measures less than 10 HU on noncontrast scan and shows a percentage washout on delayed imaging of greater than 60%.

features [70]. These lesions classically have a negative HU value caused by macroscopic fat. Because of the presence of hematopoietic tissue, the attenuation is usually higher than that of retroperitoneal fat. Areas of high attenuation that correspond to hemorrhage and calcifications may be seen as well.

Renal trauma

Renal injuries are common in patients who sustain blunt abdominal trauma. Ninety-five percent of renal injuries are minor and can be managed conservatively [71]. CT is the imaging modality of choice for evaluating blunt abdominal trauma in the hemodynamically stable patient. It can assess the severity of renal injury accurately, determine the presence of urinary extravasation and perirenal hemorrhage, and determine the status of the renal pedicle [72]. It is also an excellent modality to evaluate other nonrenal injuries. Indications for urologic imaging in patients who have blunt abdominal trauma include gross hematuria; microscopic hematuria in a hemodynamicallyunstable patient, if feasible; and microscopic hematuria associated with a positive diagnostic peritoneal lavage. Normotensive patients who have microscopic hematuria do not need any imaging, because the risk of serious injury that needs operative management in these patients is less than 0.2% [71,73,74]. The CT protocol used in evaluating renal trauma includes a corticomedullary phase at 60 to 70 seconds after injection of contrast. If the initial CT images show deep parenchymal laceration or large perirenal fluid collection [72], an excretory phase is obtained at 3 to 5 minutes after injection. Delayed scanning at 10 to 15 minutes can help assess the extent of urinary extravasation in selected patients who

are suspected of having a urine leak. If bladder rupture is suspected, then CT cystography can be added to the protocol. For the CT cystogram, at the completion of the routine trauma imaging, 50ml of 300 mgI/ml nonionic contrast (standard IV contrast) is mixed with 500cc normal saline and infused through the bladder catheter by gravity drip. The filling is continued until 400cc are instilled, or the patient becomes uncomfortable. Scanning is then performed through the pelvis. Postemptying scanning may be performed if the filled images are equivocal.

Findings on CT in patients who have renal trauma include contusion, hematoma, laceration, active bleeding, renal infarct, and urinary extravasation [73]. Renal contusion (grade I renal trauma) is characterized by a focal area of decreased enhancement in the renal parenchyma relative to normal adjacent regions, and may have sharply or poorly defined margins. Contusions are differentiated from infarcts by the absence of enhancement in the latter. Subcapsular hematomas (grade I renal trauma) may have variable attenuation values, depending on the age of the clot, with acute hematoma typically hyperattenuating (40–60 HU) relative to renal parenchyma on unenhanced CT images. Renal lacerations appear as linear, low attenuation areas in the parenchyma and may be superficial (< 1 cm depth, grade II renal trauma) or deep (> 1 cm depth, grade III renal trauma). Deep lacerations may involve the collecting system (grade IV renal trauma), which may result in urinary extravasation, diagnosed when there is contrast enhancement within a laceration or around the kidney during the excretory phase of the CT, obtained 3 to 10 minutes after contrast administration (Fig. 7). A diagnosis of traumatic false aneurysm or active hemorrhage should be considered if there

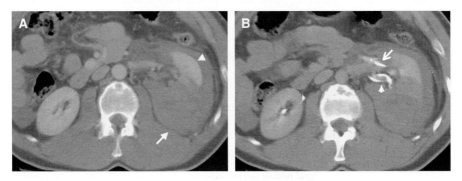

Fig. 7. Grade IV renal injury from trauma. (*A*) Venous phase with large perinephric hematoma (*arrow*) with only a small portion of the anterior cortex (*arrowhead*) preserved. (*B*) Delayed phase showing extravasation of contrast anteriorly (*arrow*) and hematoma outlined by contrast within the renal pelvis (*arrowhead*).

is intense contrast enhancement within a laceration or an adjacent hematoma during the early phase of the CT examination. In active hemorrhage, contrast tends to track into surrounding tissue and has a linear or flamelike appearance, whereas false aneurysms tend to be more focal and rounded. Patients in stable condition who have active vascular extravasation should be referred for angiographic embolization.

Thrombosis or laceration of a segmental renal arterial branch produces a focal area of renal infarction. Infarcts appear as peripherally based, wedge-shaped areas of nonenhancing renal parenchyma. Main renal artery thrombosis can lead to devascularization of the entire kidney (grade IV renal trauma). Grade V renal trauma includes shattered kidney or renal pedicle rupture. The classic findings of traumatic renal infarction at CT include absent nephrogram with retrograde opacification of the renal vein from the inferior vena cava, and abrupt truncation of the renal arterial lumen at the point of occlusion [75]. The cortical rim sign, which represents subcapsular enhancement paralleling the renal margin and is usually seen with major vascular compromise in the kidney, may be absent in the acute setting.

Genitourinary fistulas

CT is becoming increasingly useful for the diagnosis of fistulas of the genitourinary tract and is considered the primary test in some cases [76]. Although CT can be helpful in the work-up of any of the genitourinary fistulas, it is the imaging modality of choice when pyelo-alimentary, renocutaneous, and enterovesical fistulas are suspected. Parvey and colleagues [77] found that CT was the single most useful diagnostic modality for renocolic fistulas. Images can demonstrate extrarenal inflammation or an abscess extending from the kidney to the colon with complex material and gas present within the renal collecting system. In renocutaneous fistula, CT may demonstrate a soft tissue tract and surrounding inflammation, with IV contrast excreted into the affecting calyx and cutaneous tract. A sinogram may help confirm the diagnosis. CT is the primary imaging modality for suspected cases of enterovesical fistula because it may show the fistulous tract and other suggestive findings, which include intravesical air, focal bladder wall thickening, and extraluminal masses (Fig. 8). Intravesical air is a key finding and thus CT should be performed before bladder instrumentation if possible.

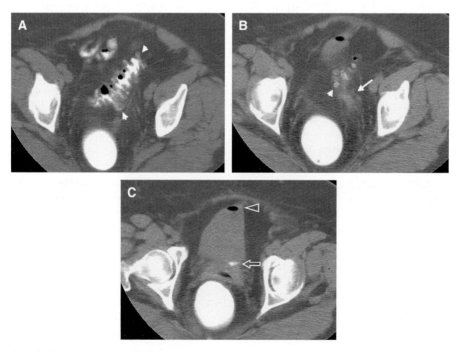

Fig. 8. Colovesical fistula from sigmoid diverticulitis. (*A*) Sigmoid colon filled with rectal contrast; numerous diverticula (*arrowheads*). (*B*) Inflammation in the fat cephalad to the sigmoid (*arrow*). (*C*) Rectal contrast (*open arrow*) and air (*open arrowhead*) both within the bladder.

Genitourinary infections

CT provides excellent anatomic details in the work-up of patients who have genitourinary infections. It is more sensitive than IVU and ultrasonography in diagnosing acute bacterial nephritis and renal and perirenal abscesses [78]. CT also improves the approach to surgical drainage and permits percutaneous approaches when used to localize renal and perirenal abscesses.

A contrast-enhanced CT scan is essential for a complete evaluation of a patient who has renal inflammatory disease, to evaluate changes in the renal parenchymal perfusion and excretion of the contrast material. The most common CT findings of acute pyelonephritis are ill-defined wedge-shaped lesions of decreased attenuation radiating from the papilla in the medulla to the cortical surface, with or without edema (Fig. 9) [21]. In immuno-compromised patients who develop emphysematous pyelonephritis, CT is the best modality for detecting the presence of gas (−150 HU or less) and for defining the extent of the disease [79].

CT is currently the most accurate modality for detecting and following renal abscesses [80]. An abscess usually appears as a well-defined low-density mass. An irregular and thick wall or pseudocapsule usually enhances on CT, whereas the liquefied purulent material does not. Gas density in a cystic mass that is fluid-filled strongly suggests abscess formation. Perinephric abscesses appear as encapsulated fluid density material within the perinephric space.

In xanthogranulomatous pyelonephritis, CT usually shows an enlarged nonfunctioning kidney that contains multiple, round, hypodense masses

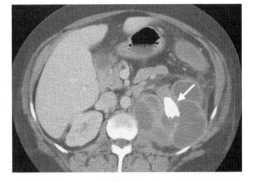

Fig. 10. Xanthogranulomatous pyelonephritis. Classic appearance of a large renal stone (*arrow*) with kidney enlarged and replaced by low attenuation masses (*bear paw sign*).

corresponding to dilated calyces or inflammatory tissue. There is usually a central calcification within the kidney (Fig. 10) [81].

Summary

Recent advances in CT imaging have made it the most commonly used imaging modality in urology and the one with which urologists are most familiar. With the introduction of CT urography, CT angiography, and 3D reconstruction, urologists are able to use a single imaging technique to perform comprehensive evaluations of patients who have different pathologies. It is thus prudent that urologists be familiar with what CT has to offer, to maximize the clinical information available to them.

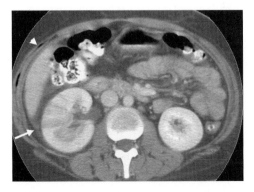

Fig. 9. Pyelonephritis. Perinephric fat stranding (*arrow*) and striated nephrogram in the right kidney. The patient was explored for appendicitis before the CT scan with residual abdominal wall air (*arrowhead*).

References

[1] Brant WE. Basic principles. In: Brant WE, Helms CA, editors. Fundamentals of diagnostic radiology. 2nd edition. Baltimore: Williams & Wilkins; 1999. p. 3–21.

[2] Lockhart ME, Smith JK. Technical considerations in renal CT. Radiol Clin North Am 2003;41(5): 863–75.

[3] Zagoria RJ. Genitourinary radiology. 2nd edition. St. Louis: CV Mosby; 2004.

[4] Bettmann MA, Heeren T, Greenfield A, et al. Adverse events with radiographic contrast agents: results of the SCVIR Contrast Agent Registry. Radiology 1997;203(3):611–20.

[5] Bettmann MA. Frequently asked questions: iodinated contrast agents. Radiographics 2004; 24(Suppl 1):S3–S10.

[6] Lasser EC, Berry CC, Talner LB, et al. Pretreatment with corticosteroids to alleviate reactions to intravenous contrast material. N Engl J Med 1987;317(14): 845–9.

[7] Rudnick MR, Goldfarb S, Wexler L, et al. Nephrotoxicity of ionic and nonionic contrast media in 1196 patients: a randomized trial. The iohexol cooperative study. Kidney Int 1995;47(1):254–61.

[8] Solomon R, Werner C, Mann D, et al. Effects of saline, mannitol, and furosemide to prevent acute decreases in renal function induced by radiocontrast agents. N Engl J Med 1994;331(21):1416–20.

[9] Tepel M, van der Giet M, Schwarzfeld C, et al. Prevention of radiographic-contrast-agent-induced reductions in renal function by acetylcysteine. N Engl J Med 2000;343(3):180–4.

[10] Chalmers N, Jackson RW. Comparison of iodixanol and iohexol in renal impairment. Br J Radiol 1999; 72(859):701–3.

[11] Aspelin P, Aubry P, Fransson SG, et al. Nephrotoxic effects in high-risk patients undergoing angiography. N Engl J Med 2003;348(6):491–9.

[12] Bailey CJ, Turner RC. Metformin. N Engl J Med 1996;334(9):574–9.

[13] Lang EK, Macchia RJ, Thomas R, et al. Improved detection of renal pathologic features on multiphasic helical CT compared with IVU in patients presenting with microscopic hematuria. Urology 2003;61(3): 528–32.

[14] Kawashima A, Vrtiska TJ, LeRoy AJ, et al. CT urography. Radiographics 2004;24(Suppl 1): S35–58.

[15] Lang EK, Macchia RJ, Thomas R, et al. Computerized tomography tailored for the assessment of microscopic hematuria. J Urol 2002;167(2 Pt 1): 547–54.

[16] Urban BA. The small renal mass: what is the role of multiphasic helical scanning? Radiology 1997; 202(1):22–3.

[17] Rydberg J, Buckwalter KA, Caldemeyer KS, et al. Multisection CT: scanning techniques and clinical applications. Radiographics 2000;20(6):1787–806.

[18] Ros PR, Ji H. Special focus session: multisection (multidetector) CT: applications in the abdomen. Radiographics 2002;22(3):697–700.

[19] Coll DM, Herts BR, Davros WJ, et al. Preoperative use of 3D volume rendering to demonstrate renal tumors and renal anatomy. Radiographics 2000;20(2): 431–8.

[20] Coll DM, Uzzo RG, Herts BR, et al. 3-Dimensional volume rendered computerized tomography for preoperative evaluation and intraoperative treatment of patients undergoing nephron sparing surgery. J Urol 1999;161(4):1097–102.

[21] Kawashima A, LeRoy AJ. Radiologic evaluation of patients with renal infections. Infect Dis Clin North Am 2003;17(2):433–56.

[22] Memarsadeghi M, Heinz-Peer G, Helbich TH, et al. Unenhanced multi-detector row CT in patients suspected of having urinary stone disease: effect of section width on diagnosis. Radiology 2005;235(2): 530–6.

[23] Smith RC, Rosenfield AT, Choe KA, et al. Acute flank pain: comparison of non-contrast-enhanced CT and intravenous urography. Radiology 1995; 194(3):789–94.

[24] Smith RC, Verga M, McCarthy S, et al. Diagnosis of acute flank pain: value of unenhanced helical CT. AJR Am J Roentgenol 1996;166(1):97–101.

[25] Miller OF, Rineer SK, Reichard SR, et al. Prospective comparison of unenhanced spiral computed tomography and intravenous urogram in the evaluation of acute flank pain. Urology 1998;52(6): 982–7.

[26] Federle MP, McAninch JW, Kaiser JA, et al. Computed tomography of urinary calculi. AJR Am J Roentgenol 1981;136(2):255–8.

[27] Schwartz BF, Schenkman N, Armenakas NA, et al. Imaging characteristics of indinavir calculi. J Urol 1999;161(4):1085–7.

[28] Dalrymple NC, Casford B, Raiken DP, et al. Pearls and pitfalls in the diagnosis of ureterolithiasis with unenhanced helical CT. Radiographics 2000;20(2): 439–47.

[29] Smith RC, Verga M, Dalrymple N, et al. Acute ureteral obstruction: value of secondary signs of helical unenhanced CT. AJR Am J Roentgenol 1996; 167(5):1109–13.

[30] Heneghan JP, Dalrymple NC, Verga M, et al. Soft-tissue "rim" sign in the diagnosis of ureteral calculi with use of unenhanced helical CT. Radiology 1997;202(3):709–11.

[31] Bell TV, Fenlon HM, Davison BD, et al. Unenhanced helical CT criteria to differentiate distal ureteral calculi from pelvic phleboliths. Radiology 1998;207(2):363–7.

[32] Rucker CM, Menias CO, Bhalla S. Mimics of renal colic: alternative diagnoses at unenhanced helical CT. Radiographics 2004;24(Suppl 1):S11–33.

[33] Chai RY, Jhaveri K, Saini S, et al. Comprehensive evaluation of patients with haematuria on multi-slice computed tomography scanner: protocol design and preliminary observations. Australas Radiol 2001; 45(4):536–8.

[34] Kopka L, Fischer U, Zoeller G, et al. Dual-phase helical CT of the kidney: value of the corticomedullary and nephrographic phase for evaluation of renal lesions and preoperative staging of renal cell carcinoma. AJR Am J Roentgenol 1997;169(6): 1573–8.

[35] Caoili EM, Cohan RH, Inampudi P, et al. MDCT urography of upper tract urothelial neoplasms. AJR Am J Roentgenol 2005;184(6):1873–81.

[36] Joffe SA, Servaes S, Okon S, et al. Multi-detector row CT urography in the evaluation of hematuria. Radiographics 2003;23(6):1441–56.

[37] McCoy JG, Honda H, Reznicek M, et al. Computerized tomography for detection and staging of

localized and pathologically defined upper tract urothelial tumors. J Urol 1991;146(6):1500–3.

[38] Scolieri MJ, Paik ML, Brown SL, et al. Limitations of computed tomography in the preoperative staging of upper tract urothelial carcinoma. Urology 2000; 56(6):930–4.

[39] McCarthy CL, Cowan NC. Multidetector CT urography (MD-CTU) for urothelial imaging [abstract]. Radiology 2002;225(P):137.

[40] Caoili EM, Coahn RH, Inampudi P, et al. MDCT urography of upper tract urothelial neoplasms. AJR Am J Roentgenol 2005;184(6):1873–81.

[41] Silverman SJ, Lee BY, Seltzer SE, et al. Small (≤ 3cm) renal masses: correlation of spiral CT features and pathologic findings. AJR Am J Roentgenol 1994;163(3):597–605.

[42] Bosniak MA, Megibow AJ, Hulnick DH, et al. CT diagnosis of renal angiomyolipoma: the importance of detecting small amounts of fat. AJR Am J Roentgenol 1988;151(3):497–501.

[43] Herts BR, Coll DM, Novick AC, et al. Enhancement characteristics of papillary renal neoplasms revealed on triphasic helical CT of the kidneys. AJR Am J Roentgenol 2002;178(2):367–72.

[44] Macari M, Bosniak MA. Delayed CT to evaluate renal masses incidentally discovered at contrast-enhanced CT: demonstration of vascularity with deenhancement. Radiology 1999;213(3):674–80.

[45] Suh M, Coakley FV, Qayyum A, et al. Distinction of renal cell carcinomas from high-attenuation renal cysts at portal venous phase contrast-enhanced CT. Radiology 2003;228(2):330–4.

[46] Bosniak MA. The current radiological approach to renal cysts. Radiology 1986;158(1):1–10.

[47] Israel GM, Bosniak MA. Calcification in cystic renal masses: is it important in diagnosis? Radiology 2003; 226(1):47–52.

[48] Bosniak MA. Diagnosis and management of patients with complicated cystic lesions of the kidney. AJR Am J Roentgenol 1997;169(3):819–21.

[49] Israel GM, Bosniak MA. An update of the Bosniak renal cyst classification system. Urology 2005;66(3): 484–8.

[50] Ratner LE, Ciseck LJ, Moore RG, et al. Laparoscopic live donor nephrectomy. Transplantation 1995;60(9):1047–9.

[51] Kawamoto S, Montgomery RA, Lawler LP, et al. Multi-detector row CT evaluation of living renal donors prior to laparoscopic nephrectomy. Radiographics 2004;24(2):453–66.

[52] Rubin GD, Alfrey EJ, Dake MD, et al. Assessment of living renal donors with spiral CT. Radiology 1995;195(2):457–62.

[53] Rydberg J, Kopecky KK, Tann M, et al. Evaluation of prospective living renal donors for laparoscopic nephrectomy with multisection CT: the marriage of minimally invasive imaging with minimally invasive surgery. Radiographics 2001;21 (Spec No):S223–36.

[54] Wang DS, Stolpen AH, Bird VG, et al. Correlation of preoperative three-dimensional magnetic resonance angiography with intraoperative findings in laparoscopic renal surgery. J Endourol 2005;19(2):193–9.

[55] Lawler LP, Jarret TW, Corl FM, et al. Adult ureteropelvic junction obstruction: insights with three-dimensional multi-detector row CT. Radiographics 2005;25(1):121–34.

[56] Martin X, Rouviere O. Radiologic evaluations affecting surgical technique in ureteropelvic junction obstruction. Curr Opin Urol 2001;11(2):193–6.

[57] Kumon H, Tsugawa M, Hashimoto H, et al. Impact of 3-dimensional helical computerized tomography on selection of operative methods for ureteropelvic junction obstruction. J Urol 1997; 158(5):1696–700.

[58] Korobkin M, Francis IR, Kloos RT, et al. The incidental adrenal mass. Radiol Clin North Am 1996; 34(5):1037–54.

[59] Renken NS, Krestin GP. Magnetic resonance imaging of the adrenal glands. Semin Ultrasound CT MR 2005;26(3):162–71.

[60] Lee MJ, Hahn PF, Papanicolaou N, et al. Benign and malignant adrenal masses: CT distinction with attenuation coefficients, size, and observer analysis. Radiology 1991;179(2):415–8.

[61] Boland GW, Lee MJ, Gazelle GS, et al. Characterization of adrenal masses using unenhanced CT: an analysis of the CT literature. AJR Am J Roentgenol 1998;171(1):201–4.

[62] Korobkin M, Brodeur FJ, Yutzy GG, et al. Differentiation of adrenal adenomas from nonadenomas using CT attenuation values. AJR Am J Roentgenol 1996;166(3):531–6.

[63] Korobkin M, Brodeur FJ, Francis IR, et al. Delayed enhanced CT for differentiation of benign from malignant adrenal masses. Radiology 1996;200(3):737–42.

[64] Boland GW, Hahn PF, Pena C, et al. Adrenal masses: characterization with delayed contrast-enhanced CT. Radiology 1997;202(3):693–6.

[65] Pena CS, Boland GW, Hahn PF, et al. Characterization of indeterminate (lipid-poor) adrenal masses: use of washout characteristics at contrast-enhanced CT. Radiology 2000;217(3):798–802.

[66] Szolar DH, Kammerhuber FH. Adrenal adenomas and nonadenomas: assessment of washout at delayed contrast-enhanced CT. Radiology 1998; 207(2):369–75.

[67] Caoili EM, Korobkin M, Francis IR, et al. Adrenal masses: characterization with combined unenhanced and delayed enhanced CT. Radiology 2002;222(3): 629–33.

[68] Korobkin M, Brodeur FJ, Francis IR, et al. CT time-attenuation washout curves of adrenal adenomas and nonadenomas. AJR Am J Roentgenol 1998;170(3):747–52.

[69] Bae KT, Fuangtharnthip P, Prasad SR, et al. Adrenal masses: CT characterization with histogram analysis method. Radiology 2003;228(3):735–42.

[70] Pereira JM, Sirlin CB, Pinto PS, et al. CT and MR imaging of extrahepatic fatty masses of the abdomen and pelvis: techniques, diagnosis, differential diagnosis, and pitfalls. Radiographics 2005;25(1): 69–85.

[71] Matthews LA, Spirnak JP. The nonoperative approach to major blunt renal trauma. Semin Urol 1995;13(1):77–82.

[72] Harris AC, Zwirewich CV, Lyburn ID, et al. CT findings in blunt renal trauma. Radiographics 2001;21(Spec No):S201–14.

[73] Miller KS, McAninch JW. Radiographic assessment of renal trauma: our 15-year experience. J Urol 1995; 154(2 Pt 1):352–5.

[74] Mee SL, McAninch JW. Indications for radiographic assessment in suspected renal trauma. Urol Clin North Am 1989;16(2):187–92.

[75] Nunez D Jr, Rivas L, McKenney K, et al. Helical CT of traumatic arterial injuries. AJR Am J Roentgenol 1998;170(6):1621–6.

[76] Yu NC, Raman SS, Patel M, et al. Fistulas of the genitourinary tract: a radiologic review. Radiographics 2004;24(5):1331–52.

[77] Parvey HR, Cochran ST, Payan J, et al. Renocolic fistulas: complementary roles of computed tomography and direct pyelography. Abdom Imaging 1997; 22(1):96–9.

[78] Soulen MC, Fishman EK, Goldman SM, et al. Bacterial renal infection: role of CT. Radiology 1989; 171(3):703–7.

[79] Wan YL, Lee TY, Bullard MJ, et al. Acute gas-producing bacterial renal infection: correlation between imaging findings and clinical outcome. Radiology 1996;198(2):433–8.

[80] Hoddick W, Jeffrey RB, Goldberg HI, et al. CT and sonography of severe renal and perirenal infections. AJR Am J Roentgenol 1983;140(3):517–20.

[81] Solomon A, Braf Z, Papo J, et al. Computerized tomography in xanthogranulomatous pyelonephritis. J Urol 1983;130(2):323–5.

ELSEVIER
SAUNDERS

Urol Clin N Am 33 (2006) 301–317

UROLOGIC
CLINICS
of North America

Understanding and Interpreting MRI of the Genitourinary Tract

Matthew J. Bassignani, MD

*Department of Radiology, University of Virginia Health Sciences Center, P.O. Box 800170,
Lee Street, Charlottesville, VA 22908, USA*

Although CT is the mainstay of cross-sectional genitourinary (GU) imaging, MRI is becoming a useful and powerful alternative for imaging the kidneys, ureters, and bladder [1,2]. In the past, MRI suffered from decreased spatial resolution when compared with CT because of long data acquisition times and degradation of images by motion. These technical limitations are being overcome gradually as imaging times become exponentially shorter and spatial resolution approaches that of CT. Contrast resolution has always been exquisite with MRI without the need for intravenous contrast administration. Three-dimensional multiplanar capabilities have also contributed to the familiar anatomic imaging of the kidneys, ureters, and bladder, which is done traditionally in the coronal plane, same as for intravenous urography. Although MRI still is considered a problem solver for issues that are not or cannot be resolved with CT, it is also a viable alternative to conventional cross-sectional imaging (ie, CT), with some important benefits.

Benefits of MRI over CT

This discussion is confined to renal mass detection and characterization. MRI can detect renal lesions on the order of 1 cm as well as CT can [3,4]; any lesion smaller than 1 cm would be difficult to characterize by either modality, and it is unlikely that a lesion this small would require immediate therapy. Staging renal lesions is more complete with MRI than CT, particularly when

determinating renal vein and inferior vena cava (IVC) involvement, which can be particularly prone to error on contrast-enhanced CT.

An increasing number of patients are being scanned with CT, and even though current nonionic, low osmolar contrast agents are generally safe, there is still a moderate adverse reaction rate of almost 1% [5]. Contrast reactions, in general, are anaphylactoid and do not represent true antibody-mediated allergic reactions. Although most contrast reactions are generally mild and self-limited, up to 25% of patients who experience one reaction will experience another after iodinated contrast readministration [6]. The potential nephrotoxicity of iodinated contrast is another drawback of CT. The contrast agent used with MRI is a chelate of the rare earth element gadolinium. In its elemental form, gadolinium is toxic, but when chelated it becomes safe, with virtually no side effects and no nephrotoxicity. Some GU patients have iodine contrast allergies or renal insufficiency, and MRI is the perfect alternative for imaging those requiring contrast (eg, for assessing a renal mass for enhancement) [7]. If nephron sparing surgery is contemplated, MRI is better able to differentiate tumor from perinephric fat, renal sinus, and collecting system, helping the urologist decide if partial nephrectomy is feasible in some patients [8]. Patients who have genetic anomalies resulting in an increased risk for renal cell carcinoma (RCCA) (eg, von Hippel-Lindau), and those with conditions that produce other renal lesions that may mimic RCCA (eg, tuberous sclerosis), can be followed safely with yearly MRI instead of CT. This follow-up regimen will protect these high-risk patients from recurrent exposure to ionizing radiation from CT, with no loss

No funding support was provided for the preparation of this article.

E-mail address: mjb4f@virginia.edu

in ability to detect or characterize renal lesions. Often, follow-up CT examinations in patients who have a history of RCCA are performed yearly. Surveillance could be performed with MRI in these patients as well. Further, the additive effects of radiation and the potential harm to developing tissues in children, or to a developing embryo in a pregnant woman, can be obviated by the use of MRI, which has shown no adverse affects in these patients. Those patients who would benefit more from renal MRI than from renal CT are as follows:

Patients with a history of iodinated contrast allergy
Patients with a compromised renal function
Children
Women of child-bearing age
Patients being considered for nephron-sparing surgery
Surveillance in patients at high risk for RCCA
Patients with a prior history of renal neoplasia who require surveillance

MRI is not for all patients. Box 1 lists the potential disadvantages of MRI over other cross-sectional imaging modalities. Patients who are critically ill (eg, ICU patients) and those who have difficulty with the breath-holding requirements of MRI are not ideal candidates. Within each MRI examination are a number of sequences geared toward answering a specific question. These sequences can be obtained within one (or more) breath holds by the patient. But the duration of each breath hold is approximately 20 to 30 seconds, and patients who are critically ill or who are unable to cooperate for other reasons

(dementia, chronic obstructive pulmonary disease, and so forth) should not have an MRI. Scanning these patients often results in a poor quality examination that may be uninterpretable. Patients who have ferromagnetic implants (neurovascular aneurysm clips, cochlear implants, pacemakers, defibrillators) cannot be placed in the magnet. Potentially, a ferromagnetic clip could move in the strong magnetic field of a magnetic resonance (MR) scanner and become dislodged from the vessel to which it is attached. Placing a pacemaker wire in a strong magnetic field can disrupt the pacemaker's normal electrical discharge and potentially lead to cardiac dysrhythmias. Examination times for MRI have shortened with the availability of stronger magnetic gradients. However, examination times at our institution are still on the order 20 to 30 minutes for a full renal mass protocol. Many patients find this amount of time in the magnet to be uncomfortable. Patients with claustrophobia may require oral sedation before the examination and even then may fail to tolerate the confined space. Experience at our institution has shown that open magnets result in significantly degraded scan quality.

Physics

In-depth physics discussions are best left to our colleagues with the slide rules. However, it is helpful to know how an image is made with MR. Patients are placed on a gantry that enters the magnetic bore of the magnet (Fig. 1). The bore,

---

Box 1. Disadvantages of MRI

MRI is not for everybody.
- Very ill, ICU patients
- Patients with pacemakers
- Patients with ferromagnetic implants
- Patients who have claustrophobia

MRI requires a longer examination time (20 to 30 minutes vs. less than 10 minutes for CT).

MRI still requires intravenous contrast administration.

Quality may be affected by variable technology and technologist experience.

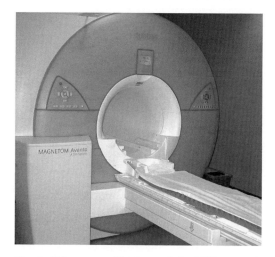

Fig. 1. MR scanner. The bore of the MRI scanner's magnet is the central opening where the strong magnetic field is generated.

which looks like a donut, produces the strong magnetic field used to create the image. In a strong magnetic field, the free water protons (ie, hydrogen ions) in the patient orient to the magnetic field, along the z-axis. The z-axis is straight through the bore, along the long axis of the patient (ie, head to toe). A radio frequency (RF) antenna, also called a "coil," is placed on the patient over the body part to be imaged. This coil transmits RF pulses through the patient and energizes the protons in the z-axis. When the RF pulses are stopped, the protons give off the energy that was imparted to them by the RF pulse. This emitted energy is received by the same RF coil and it is from this energy that the MR image is created.

Each MR sequence takes advantage of the intrinsic property of the body's tissues to absorb and give up this energy. How the energy is imparted through the physics of the pulse sequences and whether energy is released quickly or slowly determine the "weighting" of an image. In general, an image is either T1 or T2 weighted. Box 2 contains the signal intensities of common structures encountered with the T1- and T2-weighted images used in our renal neoplasm MRI protocol (Fig. 2). MRI possesses exquisite contrast resolution even without the addition of intravenous contrast. On T1-weighted images (T1WI), fluid is generally dark (also called "low signal") and on T2-weighted images (T2WI), fluid is bright (also called "high signal"). For example, within the kidney, the cortex is higher signal (or brighter) than the medulla, which is lower signal (or dark) on T1WI. On T2WI, kidneys are generally high signal because of their high fluid content. Gadolinium administration results in augmented relaxation of protons on T1WI, and thus structures that enhance with gadolinium become brighter. Box 3 lists common uses of MRI in urology.

The goal of imaging indeterminate renal cystic lesions and solid masses is to separate those lesions that should be treated surgically (eg, RCCA) from those lesions that can be characterized as benign (eg, simple cysts, angiomyolipomas (AML), complex cysts) and those lesions requiring sequential follow-up (eg, "minimal fat" AML, renal abscess, Bosniak IIF cysts). Staging of RCCA is done equally well with CT or MRI, except for the important surgical planning related to vascular invasion into renal veins or IVC [9,10]. Here, MRI outperforms CT because MRI is able to detect venous invasion with sensitivities of 100%, compared with 79% for CT [9]. In the setting of an adrenal mass, MRI can separate easily most adrenal adenomas from adrenal metastases without the need for intravenous contrast. Pheochromocytomas may be characterized more safely by MR; there are case reports of administrating iodinated contrast to patients who have pheochromocytoma resulting in a hypertensive crisis during CT. Benign adrenal masses such as myelolipomas are demonstrated well on T1WI because the fat contained within these lesions is detected easily as high signal on T1WI; the fat becomes dark with the application of a frequency-selective fat saturation pulse that nulls the signal coming from the macroscopic fat.

Renal masses

In the US, approximately 32,000 new cases of RCCA are diagnosed annually. Renal carcinoma accounts for 2% of all cancers and approximately 12,000 deaths per year [11]. More renal masses are

---

Box 2. T1- and T2-weighted image characteristics

T1-weighted image
- Simple fluid is low signal (ie, dark); internal controls: bladder, cerebrospinal fluid
- Fat is high signal (ie, bright)
- Kidneys
cortex (high signal)
medulla (low signal)

T2-weighted image
- Fluid is high signal (bright); internal controls: gallbladder, bladder, cerebrospinal fluid
- Fat is also high signal
- Kidneys
fluid (high signal)

Box 3. Common MR applications in urology

Evaluation of solid renal masses
Evaluation of renal cysts and cystic masses
Staging of RCCA
Characterization of adrenal masses

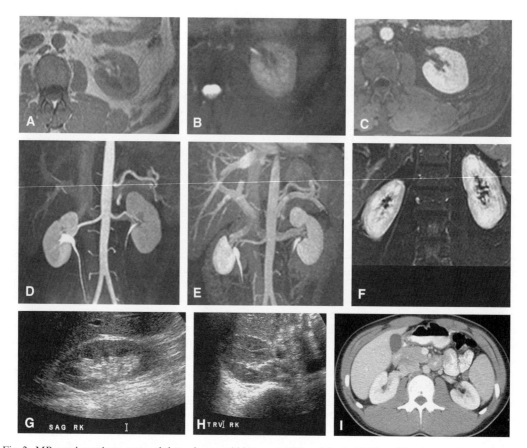

Fig. 2. MR renal neoplasm protocol through normal kidneys. (*A*) T1-weighted, (*B*) T2-weighted, and (*C*) T1 postgadolinium image (last two with fat saturation). (*D*) MR angiogram and (*E*) MR venogram of abdominal vascular in coronal plane. (*F*) Subtraction images of kidneys in coronal plane. Ultrasound of normal kidneys in (*G*) sagittal and (*H*) transverse planes. (*I*) CT with intravenous iodinated contrast of normal kidneys in axial plane.

being detected in asymptomatic patients because of the expanded use of imaging for myriad reasons. MRI is equivalent to CT in ability to detect renal lesions of approximately 1 cm [3,4], and in detecting lymphadenopathy [12]. MR detects polar lesions more often and it outperforms CT in correctly diagnosing venous invasion (100% sensitivity).

Our renal mass protocol includes the sequences shown in Table 1. Box 4 lists the uses of each sequence for renal lesion detection and characterization; evaluation for adenopathy; and detection of renal vein and IVC invasion.

The signal characteristics within a renal mass detected by MRI correlate well to findings on pathologic examination [3]. For example, high signal on T1WI may represent areas of hemorrhage, necrosis, or proteinaceous debris within a renal mass. Enhancing elements represent viable tumor

(Fig. 3). On T2WI, renal lesions are often higher signal than the surrounding normal renal parenchyma, making them more conspicuous (Fig. 4). The most important factor in determining if a renal lesion is a solid neoplasm is the presence of enhancement. Enhancement is evaluated by comparing unenhanced T1WI to gadolinium-enhanced T1WI; any detectable lesion is assessed for perceivable or measurable increase in signal intensity after contrast. Qualitative assessment of enhancement is a reasonable approach to diagnosing an enhancing renal mass. If the lesion is brighter in the postcontrast images than in the precontrast images, it is safe to conclude it is enhancing (Fig. 5). A quantitative approach espoused by Ho and colleagues [13] is to measure regions of interest (ROI) within the lesion precontrast and after administration of gadolinium. With all other scan parameters held constant

Table 1
Renal neoplasm MRI protocol sequences

Sequence	Plane	TR (ms)	TE (ms)	Flip Angle	Thickness (mm)	Gap (mm)
T2 HASTE	Cor	1000	80.0	180	5.0	0.0
T2 HASTE	Ax	1000	75.0	180	5.0	0.0
T1 Gradient Echo	Ax	128	4.8	70	5.0	0.1
T1 Gradient Echo (FS)	Ax	135	4.8	70	5.0	0.1
Dynamic T1 3D Gradient Echo (FS)	Ax	3.73	1.7	12	2.5	0.0
Turbo MRA	Cor	2.89	1.1	20	Variable	0.0

Abbreviations: Ax, axial; FS, fat saturation; HASTE, half-Fourier acquisition single-shot turbo spin-echo; Cor, coronal; Sag, sagittal; TE, echo time; the time from the start of the pulse sequence until the signal (ie, the echo) is acquired; TR, repetition time; the time between successive pulse sequences; Turbo MRA, magnetic resonance angiography rapid acquisition examination following administration of intravenous gadolinium.

between the pre- and postcontrast images, if the lesion increases in signal intensity by more than 15%, then the lesion is said to be enhancing, indicating a solid renal neoplasm (Fig. 6). Percentage of enhancement is calculated as follows: $[(SI_{post} - SI_{pre})/SI_{pre}] \times 100\%$, where SI_{pre} is the precontrast signal intensity of the lesion and SI_{post} is the postcontrast signal intensity of the lesion. On T2WI, foci of signal as high as the signal from cerebrospinal fluid, for example, represent areas of fluid or cystic change (Fig. 7).

Benign lesions such as AML also enhance. However, T1WI with MRI will detect the high signal fat contained within these renal lesions accurately. With fat saturation sequences, the fatty portions of the mass drop in signal, which is diagnostic of a fat-containing renal mass, virtually pathognomonic for AML (Fig. 8). After the exclusion of AML, and in the absence of lymphoma and metastatic disease, all other enhancing renal lesions represent surgical lesions. Unfortunately, neither CT nor MRI can differentiate oncocytomas from RCCA. Box 5 lists the imaging characteristics of RCCA.

Renal cysts

Renal cysts are common. Although it is rare for patients younger than 30 years old to have cysts, renal cysts increase with age. It is common to detect renal cysts in patients over the age of 50. Acquired cystic disease of dialysis is encountered frequently in tertiary care settings. Patients who have inherited cystic diseases are followed routinely by urologists or nephrologists for close surveillance of their kidneys. Approximately 15% of all RCCAs are partly cystic [14]. Morton Bosniak, a uroradiologist, developed a systematic method to help differentiate benign renal cysts from cystic renal neoplasms, using CT criteria. There is a significant correlation between CT and MRI when applying the Bosniak system, and MRI is an equally useful tool for assessing whether a renal cyst is harboring a malignancy. Cyst characteristics on MRI are listed in Box 6.

Box 4. Renal neoplasm MRI protocol sequences and uses

T2 HASTE
- It is rapidly acquired.
- It provides good anatomy overview.
- Fluid-containing structures are bright.

T1 gradient echo
- Fat is bright (AML and myelolipomas are conspicuous).
- Complex fluid (eg, hemorrhage) is also bright.
- Adenopathy is easily visualized.

T1 gradient echo with fat saturation
- Fat-containing structures become dark.
- Complex fluid remains bright.

T1 gradient echo 3D dynamic sequence (after intravenous administration of gadolinium)
- Enhancement within any portions of a mass or cyst is consistent with a neoplasm.
- Vessels enhance.

MR angiography and MR venography
- Vessels enhance, allowing for detection of renal vein and IVC involvement.
- Vascular anatomy can be mapped.

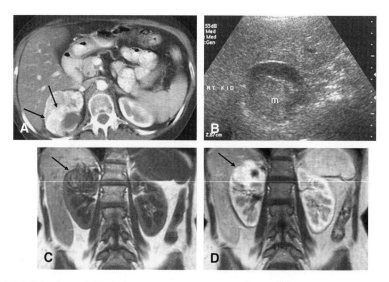

Fig. 3. RCCA. (*A*) Axial enhanced CT shows right upper pole enhancing renal mass (*arrows*). (*B*) Ultrasound correlation to CT shows mass (*m*). (*C*) T1-weighted coronal MRI shows right upper pole renal mass (*arrow*). (*D*) T1 postgadolinium fat saturation image shows intensely enhancing mass (*arrow*).

Simple cysts have characteristic imaging findings on ultrasound, CT, and MRI. With ultrasound, renal cysts are described as being anechoic, being round or oval, having an imperceptibly thin wall, and producing acoustic enhancement. With CT, simple cysts are round or oval and have a thin wall, with no perceptible internal contents. The fluid in these lesions should have the same attenuation measurement as simple fluid (less than 20 Hounsfield units). Unenhanced and enhanced imaging are required to ensure the cystic lesion does not possess enhancing components in the wall or septa. Characteristic findings on MRI mimic those on CT. These round or oval lesions follow the signal intensity of simple fluid on all sequences and therefore are low signal on T1WI and high signal on T2WI. No internal structures should be appreciable, neither wall thickening nor septa.

After gadolinium there is no enhancement seen in the cyst. Simple cysts are believed to arise from obstructed collecting tubules (Fig. 9) [15]. These lesions require no further work-up.

Complex cysts are essentially simple cysts with an added layer of complexity. Processes that may complicate an otherwise simple cyst include hemorrhage, infection, or debris, which results in variable signal on T1- and T2WI. Hemorrhage often result in high signal on T1WI because of the paramagnetic effects of blood breakdown products [16]. Proteinaceous contents within a cyst may also yield high signal on T1WI. On T2WI, older hemorrhage may result in a black ring along the cyst wall from deposition of old blood (methemoglobin) or the entire cyst may be low signal (dark). Hairline septa and thin eggshell-like calcifications may be seen within the cyst. MRI has an enhanced ability to detect cyst septa, when

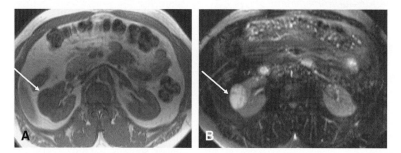

Fig. 4. RCCA. (*A*) T1-weighted axial MRI shows hypointense (dark) right midpole renal mass (*arrow*). (*B*) T2-weighted axial image shows hyperintense (bright) renal mass (*arrow*).

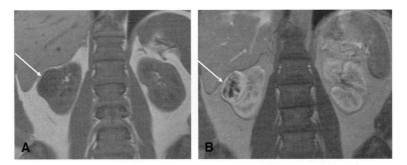

Fig. 5. RCCA. (*A*) T1-weighted coronal MRI shows hypointense right midpole renal mass (*arrow*). (*B*) T1-weighted postgadolinium coronal image shows enhancing renal mass (*arrow*).

compared with CT [17]. No enhancement should be observed in any component of the complex cyst. On CT, high density lesions of less than 3 cm, which show no enhancement, fall into the category of Bosniak II complex cysts (Fig. 10).

These lesions generally require no further work-up.

MRI is insensitive to calcification detection. This characteristic originally was thought to represent a downside to MRI when assessing

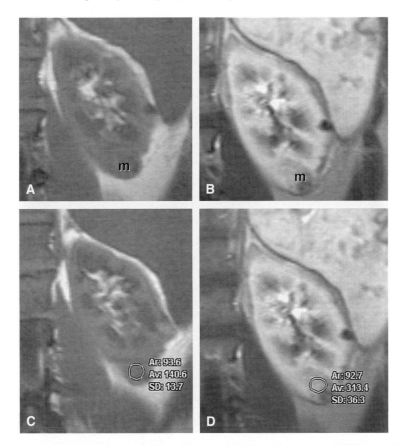

Fig. 6. Calculation of percentage enhancement in renal mass. (*A*) T1-weighted coronal MRI shows hypointense left lower pole renal mass (*m*). (*B*) T1-weighted postgadolinium coronal image shows the mass to be enhancing (*m*). (*C*) Same image as in (*A*), with region of interest drawn over renal mass, showing an average signal intensity of 141. (*D*) Same image as in (*B*), with region of interest drawn over enhancing renal mass, showing an average signal intensity of 313. Percentage enhancement is calculated at 122%, verifying enhancement in this RCCA.

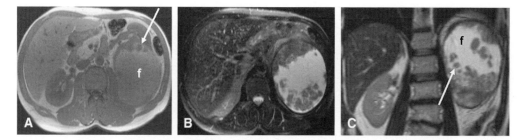

Fig. 7. Cystic RCCA. Several images show solid components within a large cystic mass. (*A*) T1-weighted axial image shows large left renal mass that is predominantly cystic, containing complex fluid (note high signal fluid (*f*); nodules within the mass represent the solid component of this neoplasm (*arrows*). (*B*) T2-weighted fat saturation axial image shows high signal intensity to the cystic fluid (*f*). (*C*) T2-weighted coronal image shows same fluid (*f*) components and nodules (*arrows*) as in (*A*).

renal cystic lesions. However, Israel, Bosniak, and colleagues [18] studied calcifications as an independent risk factor for renal carcinoma and determined that, in general, the presence of calcifications is the less predictive finding of RCCA in renal cysts, when compared with the finding of enhancement within portions of the cyst. On CT, calcification actually may produce a beam-hardening artifact that can hamper the radiologist's ability to measure enhancement within solid portions of the cyst. Therefore, MRI may be considered the preferred method to assess calcified cysts because the calcification does not interfere with ability to perceive and measure contrast enhancement.

A beam-hardening artifact may result in false attenuation measurements on CT, leading to the spurious assessment of enhancement within a renal lesion. The artifact can be seen also with small simple cysts that are surrounded by intensely enhancing renal parenchyma during the dynamic (ie, enhanced) phase of a CT scan; this artifact is known as renal "pseudoenhancement." An elegant experiment was performed to determine why some simple cysts appear to enhance after contrast but, pathologically, are proven to be simple cysts [19]. Researchers placed water-filled balloons in baths containing various concentrations of iodinated contrast. The water balloons surrounded by higher concentrations of iodinated contrast gave measurements that were higher attenuation than those of simple water. This apparent enhancement was termed pseudoenhancement and represents a combination of the beam-hardening artifact and the image-reconstruction algorithm used by the CT scanner. The pertinent clinical example is when a simple cyst attenuation

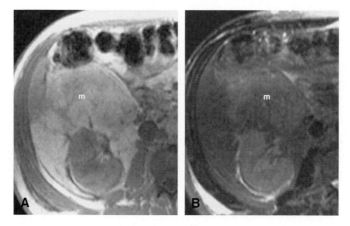

Fig. 8. Other renal masses. (*A*) T1-weighted and (*B*) T2-weighted axial fat saturation images show fatty mass (*m*) arising from anterior aspect of the right upper kidney. With fat saturation in (*B*), the mass loses signal (ie, becomes dark), consistent with a fatty mass. Diagnosis is angiomyolipoma.

Box 5. RCCA characteristics on MRI

- Imaging characteristics of tumor correlate well with gross pathology.
- T1WI is usually isointense (same signal as kidney) or hypointense (dark), but highly variable because of signal from necrosis or hemorrhage.
- T2WI is variable, but usually slightly hyperintense (bright).
- With gadolinium, tumor enhances, but less than normal renal parenchyma.
- Enhancement represents viable tumor.
- Lack of enhancement suggests necrosis or cystic formation.

Box 6. Cyst characteristics on MRI

Bosniak I (simple cysts)
- Hypointense (dark) on T1WI
- Hyperintense (bright) on T2WI
- No internal structures
- No enhancement

Bosniak II (complex cysts)
- Hypointense (dark) or hyperintense (bright) on T1WI (ie, variable signal)
- Variable on T2WI
- "Hairline" thin (< 1mm) septa
- Eggshell calcifications
- No enhancement

Bosniak III (indeterminate cysts)
- Variable T1 signal
- Variable T2 signal, but usually hyperintense (bright) signal
- Smooth or irregular septa with enhancement or smooth or irregular wall thickening with enhancement

Bosniak IV (cystic RCCA)
- Variable T1 signal
- Variable T2 signal, but usually hyperintense (bright) signal
- Solid components demonstrating measurable enhancement
- Mural nodularity
- Smooth or irregular wall thickening
- Smooth or irregular septa

Bosniak IIF (F for follow up)
- Variable signal intensities
- Questionable enhancing elements
- Many septa
- Chunky (masslike) calcification

---

is measured precontrast and after contrast administration; pseudoenhancement artifact results in measurably higher attenuation of the cyst on the enhanced portion of the scan. This finding may lead to the false conclusion that the cyst is enhancing, and thus may represent a neoplasm. To account for the variations in attenuation of renal cysts by CT, at our institution a renal lesion must enhance by more than 20 Hounsfield units to be considered truly enhancing, with a threshold of 15 Hounsfield units considered "borderline" enhancement [20]. MRI, again, is not subject to this type of artifact and thus MRI can be used as a problem solver in this circumstance.

High density cysts, defined as cysts that have a higher CT density than the adjacent nonenhanced parenchyma, represent still another kind of complex cyst. To differentiate between a high density cyst (no enhancement seen) and a high density cystic renal mass (where enhancement is present), intravenous contrast administration is required (Figs. 10 and 11). Often, high density cysts will be complex on MRI, possibly showing high signal intensity on T1WI related to hemorrhage or proteinaceous debris within the cyst. After gadolinium, enhancing lesions would also appear high signal intensity. To determine if the high signal intensity is related to enhancement in the cyst or to complex high signal fluid, we use a technique called subtraction. On the scanner, the technologist postprocesses pregadolinium and postgadolinium T1WI images, whereby the unenhanced T1WI scan is subtracted mathematically from the enhanced T1WI. If signal is still present in the cyst after subtraction, then elements within the cyst are truly enhancing (Fig. 12).

Bosniak III lesions are known as indeterminate cysts. These cysts will show variable signal on T1- and T2WI. These lesions contain thickened, irregular or smooth septa or wall showing measurable enhancement. Cystic lesions with large calcifications also are placed in this category. Fig. 13 shows an indeterminate, Bosniak III type cyst. These lesions require surgical exploration.

Bosniak IV lesions are frank cystic RCCAs and demonstrate enhancing solid components within a predominantly cystic lesion. Elements that enhance may include portions of the cyst wall,

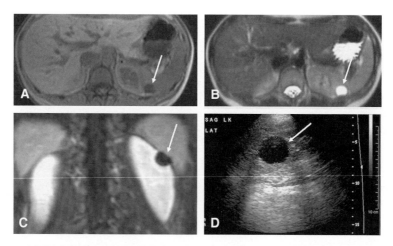

Fig. 9. Simple cyst. (*A*) T1-weighted axial, (*B*) T2-weighted axial, and (*C*) T1-weighted postgadolinium fat saturation coronal images show a simple cyst in left upper renal pole (*arrow*). (*D*) Ultrasound correlation shows a round cyst (*arrow*) with simple characteristics of imperceptible thin wall, anechoic (black) center, and increased sound through transmission behind the cyst wall.

a mural nodule, or thick septation within the cyst. Fig. 14 shows a cystic RCCA, Bosniak IV.

The Bosniak classification itself becomes complex. Bosniak realized that some cysts do not fall easily into category II or III, making the decision between surgical treatment and observation not clear cut. Thus, he created a category IIF (for follow-up) [21]. These lesions may be slightly more complex than a Bosniak type II renal cyst, but not so complex that immediate surgery is

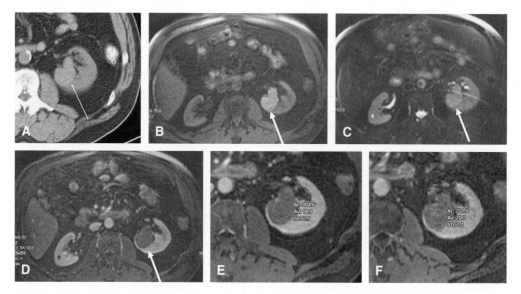

Fig. 10. Complex cyst. (*A*) Unenhanced axial CT scan through left upper kidney shows a 3-cm-high density mass or cyst (*arrow*). Because the patient had renal insufficiency, MRI was performed for further characterization. (*B*) T1-weighted axial fat saturation image shows that the lesion does not follow signal characteristics of simple fluid (ie, it is not dark on T1WI). (*C*) T2-weighted axial fat saturation image shows the lesion is fluid containing (ie, it is high signal like cerebrospinal fluid). (*D*) T1-weighted axial postgadolinium fat saturation MRI image shows no enhancement, confirming this to be a complex renal cyst (Bosniak II). (*E*) Axial T1-weighted fat saturation in early phase of gadolinium administration shows the lesion measures 18 mean signal intensity units. (*F*) Later phase of gadolinium administration shows the lesion measures 20 mean signal intensity units. Enhancement for this lesion is 11%, representing no significant enhancement.

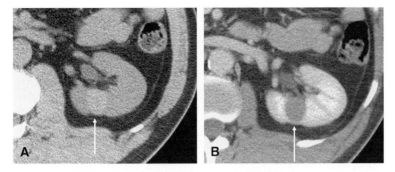

Fig. 11. Hyperdense cyst. (*A*) Axial unenhanced CT image shows a high density left midpole renal cyst or mass (*arrow*). (*B*) After iodinated contrast administration, the lesion had no appreciable change in attenuation, consistent with a complex renal cyst (Bosniak II).

warranted. These are the "watchful waiting" kidney lesions that can be followed closely in a reliable patient. If the lesion becomes more complex, it will declare itself as a Bosniak III or IV, thus requiring surgery. However, if the lesion remains stable, it may be followed safely without change for years. Those patients who are poor operative candidates, or who succumb to intercurrent illnesses before a small lesion becomes clinically important, may be followed as well, with their treatment options reassessed at follow-up [22]. Some Bosniak IIF lesions actually may become less complex over time and thus require no further work-up (eg, hemorrhagic cyst, which becomes simple appearing once the hemorrhagic clot resorbs).

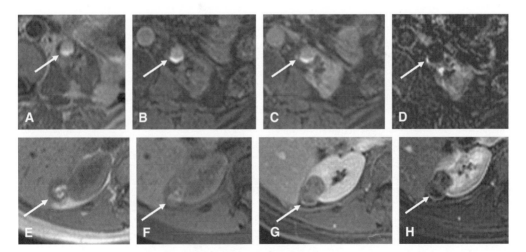

Fig. 12. Subtraction images in two different subjects. Subject 1 shows a complex cystic lesion in left midpole (*arrow*) on (*A*) T1WI, (*B*) T1WI with fat saturation, (*C*) T1WI after gadolinium and (*D*) subtraction images. Please note that it would be difficult to discern if the high signal on postgadolinium images (*C*) is due to baseline high signal, as seen in (*A*) and (*B*), or if it represents true enhancement. However, subtraction images, whereby the signal present on the initial image is subtracted from the postgadolinium image, show only what has changed between these two sequences. Note that there is no signal within the cyst on subtraction image (*D*), consistent with a nonenhancing cyst. The opposite is true for subject 2. A complex cystic lesion in right midpole (*arrow*) is seen on (*E*) T1WI, (*F*) T1WI with fat saturation, (*G*) T1WI after gadolinium, and (*H*) subtraction images. Note that on the subtraction images (*H*), there is obvious signal within the cystic lesion, representing the enhancement that occurred in this cystic renal neoplasm after gadolinium administration.

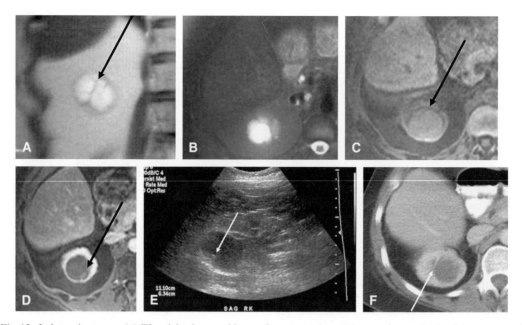

Fig. 13. Indeterminate cyst. (*A*) T2-weighted coronal image shows septa (*arrow*) in a cystic mass in the right upper renal pole. (*B*) T2-weighted axial image with fat saturation. (*C*) T1-weighted axial image with fat saturation shows no drop in signal, demonstrating no fat in the mass. (*D*) After gadolinium, the septa show enhancement (*arrow*). (*E*) Ultrasound showing same cyst with septation (*arrow*). (*F*) Contrast-enhanced CT obtained for other reasons also shows the septation (*arrow*).

Renal cell CA staging

Tumor, nodes, and metastasis (TNM) staging is becoming the preeminent staging system for RCCA [23]. With refinement over the years, it has shown a greater prognostic value than the formerly popular Robson staging system. Once a lesion is shown to enhance on MRI, RCCA is the primary consideration, and staging of the tumor can be performed with the images acquired during the MR examination. With TNM staging, T, for tumor, is determined, based on the maximal size of the tumor, measured along the tumor's long axis. Volumetric (ie, 3D) data sets in CT and MRI make this measurement easy to perform, and the longest dimension of the tumor should be reported to allow for accurate T staging of the renal neoplasm. Nodal disease is characterized equally well with MRI as with CT. By convention, pathologic nodes are those nodes measuring more than 1 cm in short axis. Lymph nodes are intermediate in signal on T1WI, similar in signal intensity to muscle. Nodes are seen best on T1WI because they stand out against the background of abdominal and retroperitoneal fat, which is very bright on T1WI (Fig. 15). Renal mass invasion into adjacent structures, such as the liver or psoas muscle,

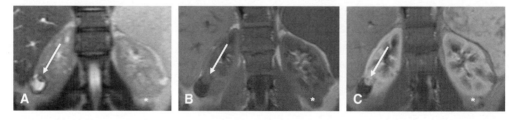

Fig. 14. Cystic RCCA. Coronal (*A*) T2-weighted, (*B*) T1-weighted pregadolinium, and (*C*) T1-weighted postgadolinium images show a cystic lesion in the lower pole of the right kidney containing a mural nodule (*arrow*) that enhances after gadolinium administration. Did you notice the left lower pole enhancing solid mass (*), representing a second RCCA in this patient who has von Hippel-Lindau?

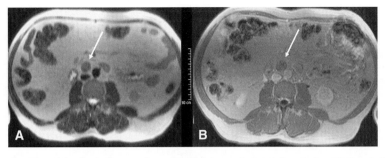

Fig. 15. Adenopathy. T1-weighted axial images through midabdomen before (*A*) and after (*B*) the administration of gadolinium shows aortocaval lymph node enlargement (*arrow*) from metastatic disease.

and distant metastatic deposits can be assessed with T1WI before and after gadolinium enhancement (Fig. 16). MRI outperforms CT when evaluating tumor invasion into the renal vein or IVC, with negative predictive values of nearly 100% for the absence of tumor involvement (Fig. 17) [24]. All sequences in the MRI provide some information about the patency of the vascular structures, but flow-sensitive techniques are used specifically to assess for vascular invasion. Gadolinium-enhanced MR arteriography and MR venography provide exquisite arterial and venous mapping and determine more accurately the extent of any thrombus, compared with CT. Arterial and venous anatomy are well shown, including anomalies such as duplicated renal arteries and circumaortic and retroaortic renal veins, further assisting the urologist with surgical planning.

Adrenal imaging

Many people find adrenal imaging confusing because of the multitude of ways in which an adrenal mass can be imaged. Imaging is brought to bear when an adrenal lesion in a patient who has cancer may represent a metastasis; when a patient has markers for pheochromocytoma; or when an otherwise healthy individual has an incidentally discovered adrenal mass. When an incidental adrenal mass is found during the staging work-up of a patient who has cancer but no other identified or suspected metastatic disease, an important part of staging involves excluding an adrenal metastasis. This analysis is handled best with CT, which can diagnose adrenal adenoma accurately with specificities close to 100% [25]. In cases that cannot be characterized by CT, or for patients who have a contraindication to iodinated contrast, adrenal MRI may be done with equal accuracy in diagnosing adrenal adenomas [26]. Benign adrenal adenomas contain a significant amount of lipid in their cytoplasm. The lipid is the precursor to the steroid hormones synthesized by the adrenal cortex. Metastases do not contain significant lipid in their cytoplasm [26]. MRI uses an artifact known as chemical shift to identify

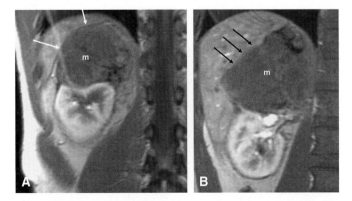

Fig. 16. Hepatic invasion. T1-weighted coronal postgadolinium MR images show a large right upper pole renal mass (*m*). (*A*) Sharp demarcation is seen between liver and renal mass on this image (*white arrows*). (*B*) No clear demarcation between the renal mass and the liver is seen on a more anterior image, representing hepatic invasion by the mass (*black arrows*).

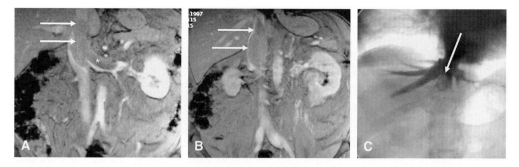

Fig. 17. Venous invasion. Coronal T1-weighted postgadolinium MR images (*A*) and (*B*) show thrombus in left renal vein (*) and IVC (*arrows*) extending just below the heart. (*C*) Hepatic venogram shows filling defect in IVC (*arrow*) just below the heart.

benign lipid-containing adrenal adenomas [27]. Chemical shift artifact occurs when approximately equal amounts of lipid and water are in the volume being imaged. The signals of these two components cancel one another out when chemical shift is maximized. Thus, the lipid-sensitive sequence actually is performed in two separate sequences of one scan. In one sequence, known as "in-phase," chemical shift artifact is at a minimum and the signals of lipid and water are additive. In the second sequence, known as "opposed-phase," chemical shift artifact is at a maximum, and the signals of lipid and water cancel one another, resulting in the adrenal mass being darker on the opposed-phase images when visually or quantitatively compared with the in-phase images (Fig. 18). CT is the test of choice in assessing potential adrenal adenomas. When CT is equivocal, MRI may be used [28].

In the proper clinical setting of elevated urinary metanephrines or elevated resting plasma catecholamines, MRI can be performed to locate pheochromocytomas, which have relatively reliable imaging characteristics [29]. A screening MR scan is performed from the level of the adrenal glands, where approximately 90% of pheochromocytomas are found. The scan continues through the paraspinal region (along the sympathetic chain) and down through the region of the organ of Zuckerkandl to the bladder dome using T2WI in-phase, and T1WI opposed-phase, and T1 pre- and postgadolinium imaging with fat-selective saturation techniques. Pheochromocytomas present as high signal masses on T2WI and often enhance intensely after gadolinium administration. Pheochromocytomas, in general, do not drop in signal on opposed-phase imaging. Myelolipoma is a fat-containing lesion that originates from the adrenal gland and is diagnosed easily with CT and MRI. It is often difficult to determine if a large fat-containing lesion has arisen from the adrenal gland, or if it is primarily a retroperitoneal mass with mass effect on, or invasion of, the adrenal gland, such as a retroperitoneal liposarcoma.

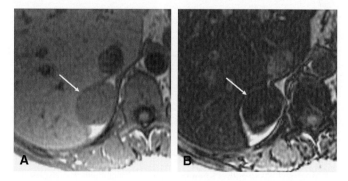

Fig. 18. Adrenal adenoma. T1-weighted gradient echo axial images of right adrenal mass (*arrow*) using in-phase (*A*) and opposed-phase (*B*) sequences shows drop-out of signal (ie, adrenal mass gets darker) on opposed-phased sequence, consistent with adrenal adenoma.

If the lesion's origin from the adrenal gland cannot be confirmed, the mass should be followed closely to assess for rapid growth. Rapid growth or pain is an indication to remove the retroperitoneal fatty mass because it raises the possibility of a liposarcoma. The remaining adrenal lesions require a tailored approach. There are no specific findings in primary adrenal carcinoma, although often they are described as large lesions, being more than 6 cm at diagnosis. Biopsy of primary adrenal carcinoma is often unhelpful in the diagnosis. Usually, primary resection is undertaken if adrenal adenoma cannot be confirmed by imaging studies.

MR urography and advanced techniques

MR urography (MRU) is an alternative to conventional intravenous urography and CT urography. Because the spatial resolution of MRU is limited when assessing the calyces, infundibuli, renal pelvis, and ureters, MRU is best reserved for when patients cannot undergo intravenous urography or CT urography. MRU uses one or both of the following techniques: heavily T2-weighted images, which show fluid-containing structures as bright; or gadolinium-enhanced excretory MRU, whereby excreted gadolinium opacifies the collecting systems.

A combination of these two techniques provides complementary information. Heavily T2-weighted coronal sequences can be performed with consecutive thin slices (4 mm) that provide fine detail (Fig. 19A). Coronal thick slabs (4 cm or more) performed in multiple obliquities provide a global overview of the collecting systems (Fig. 19B). Heavily T2-weighted sequences take advantage of the high fluid content of urine-containing structures, with urine acting as an intrinsic contrast agent. This fluid appears as very bright signal on the T2-weighted images obtained. Normal findings include high signal fluid throughout the nondilated calyces, infundibuli, renal pelvis, ureters, and bladder. If caliectasis or ureterectasis is identified, the cause and level of obstruction are sought (Fig. 20). Obstruction from stricture, extrinsic compression, or filling defects can be assessed without intravenous contrast administration. Filling defects in the fluid may represent stones, tumor, blood clot, sloughed papilla, or fungus balls. Periureteral edema suggests an acutely obstructing stone as the cause for hydroureteronephrosis. A limitation of this technique is the lack of renal functional information (ie, the technique images the fluid already present in the collecting system). Inadequate distension of the collecting system limits ability to visualize abnormalities. Wall thickening from inflammation or from transitional cell carcinoma might be

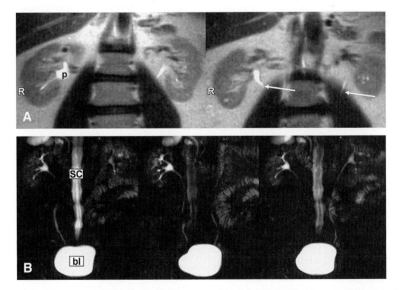

Fig. 19. (*A*) Thin slice MR urogram. Consecutive 5-mm slices from T2-weighted coronal images show fine detail of the renal pelvis (*p*) and proximal ureters (*arrows*). (*B*) Thick slab MR urogram. Consecutive 4-cm-thick slab T2-weighted coronal image obtained in three separate obliquities shows global overview of nonobstructed calyces, infundibuli, renal pelves, ureters, and bladder (*bl*). These 4-cm coronal slabs also include portions of the spinal canal (*SC*).

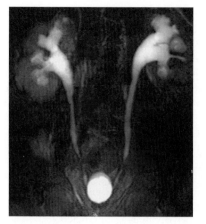

Fig. 20. Thick slab MR urogram. Four-cm-thick slab T2-weighted coronal image shows dilated collecting systems bilaterally down to the level of the bladder. Collecting system dilation was due to bladder wall thickening from muscular hypertrophy.

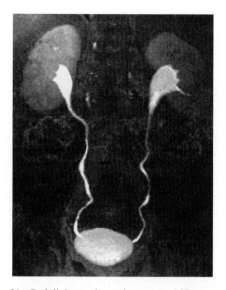

Fig. 21. Gadolinium-enhanced excretory MR urogram. Coronal T1WI with fat saturation after intravenous gadolinium administration shows excreted contrast filling nondilated collecting systems, ureters, and bladder.

visualized inadequately. Calcifications in stones may not be seen with MRI even though the filling defect and obstruction will be evident.

Gadolinium-enhanced excretory MRU is performed using T1WI with fat saturation obtained as a volume acquisition (3D) in the coronal plane. Normal findings include uptake and excretion of the high signal (ie, bright) contrast into nondilated collecting systems (Fig. 21). With intravenous gadolinium administration, kidney function can be assessed, in addition to the morphology of the collecting systems. These sequences show ureteral wall thickening and abnormal enhancement, suggesting tumor or inflammation. These sequences also show strictures, extrinsic compression, or filling defects in the excreted contrast column. Limitations of this technique include poor excretion of contrast, caused by renal obstruction or renal insufficiency. For both techniques, adequate hydration is essential and intravenous furosemide administration may be required to achieve adequate urinary distension. Gadolinium and furosemide will not distend the collecting systems adequately in patients who have chronic renal insufficiency and atrophic kidneys.

A detailed discussion of advanced techniques such as MRU [30,31], MR of bladder carcinoma [32], and MR spectroscopy for prostate cancer [33,34] is beyond the space constraints of this article. The reader is referred to the many informative articles about these techniques.

Summary

MRI has evolved slowly into a useful imaging tool for GU patients who cannot have iodinated contrast, for patients who require a problem-solving modality for equivocal ultrasound or CT findings, or for those patients for whom repeated CT may represent an unacceptable exposure to ionizing radiation. Still, MRI is not for all patients because the scan time remains relatively prolonged when compared with CT. Some patients cannot be scanned with MRI due to absolute (pacemaker, other ferromagnetic implants) or relative (claustrophobia) contraindications. MRI is a sophisticated procedure that requires substantial technical and medical expertise for performing the examination and interpreting findings. Close communication between the urologist and the uroradiologist is required to determine if MR imaging of the GU system is right for a particular patient.

Acknowledgments

The author wishes to thank Dr. William Brant and Dr. Ruth Moran for manuscript editing assistance, and Shirley Naylor and Sherry Deane for assistance with the preparation of this manuscript.

References

[1] Farres MT, Gattegno B, Ronco P, et al. Nonnephro-toxic, dynamic, contrast enhanced magnetic resonance urography: use in nephrology and urology. J Urol. Apr 2000;163(4):1191–6 quiz 1295.

[2] Probert JL, Glew D, Gillatt DA. Magnetic resonance imaging in urology. BJU Int 1999;83(3):201–14.

[3] Pretorius ES, Wickstrom ML, Siegelman ES. MR imaging of renal neoplasms. Magn Reson Imaging Clin N Am 2000;8(4):813–36.

[4] Semelka RC, Hricak H, Stevens SK, et al. Combined gadolinium-enhanced and fat-saturation MR imaging of renal masses. Radiology 1991;178(3):803–9.

[5] Thomsen HS, Bush WH Jr. Adverse effects of contrast media: incidence, prevention and management. Drug Saf 1998;19(4):313–24.

[6] Bettmann MA, Heeren T, Greenfield A, et al. Adverse events with radiographic contrast agents: results of the SCVIR Contrast Agent Registry. Radiology 1997;203(3):611–20.

[7] Rudnick MR, Berns JS, Cohen RM, et al. Contrast media-associated nephrotoxicity. Semin Nephrol 1997;17(1):15–26.

[8] Pretorius ES, Siegelman ES, Ramchandani P, et al. Renal neoplasms amenable to partial nephrectomy: MR imaging. Radiology 1999;212(1):28–34.

[9] Kallman DA, King BF, Hattery RR, et al. Renal vein and inferior vena cava tumor thrombus in renal cell carcinoma: CT, US, MRI and venacavography. J Comput Assist Tomogr 1992;16(2):240–7.

[10] Oto A, Herts BR, Remer EM, et al. Inferior vena cava tumor thrombus in renal cell carcinoma: staging by MR imaging and impact on surgical treatment. AJR Am J Roentgenol 1998;171(6):1619–24.

[11] Greenlee RT, Hill-Harmon MB, Murray T, et al. Cancer statistics, 2001. CA Cancer J Clin 2001;51(1):15–36.

[12] Hricak H, Thoeni RF, Carroll PR, et al. Detection and staging of renal neoplasms: a reassessment of MR imaging. Radiology 1988;166(3):643–9.

[13] Ho VB, Allen SF, Hood MN, et al. Renal masses: quantitative assessment of enhancement with dynamic MR imaging. Radiology 2002;224(3):695–700.

[14] Hartman DS, Davis CJ Jr, Johns T, et al. Cystic renal cell carcinoma. Urology 1986;28(2):145–53.

[15] Grantham JJ, Winklhofer F. Brenner & Rector's the kidney. 6th edition. Philadelphia: W.B. Saunders Company; 2000.

[16] Roubidoux MA. MR imaging of hemorrhage and iron deposition in the kidney. Radiographics 1994;14(5):1033–44.

[17] Israel GM, Hindman N, Bosniak MA. Evaluation of cystic renal masses: comparison of CT and MR imaging by using the Bosniak classification system. Radiology 2004;231(2):365–71.

[18] Israel GM, Bosniak MA. Calcification in cystic renal masses: is it important in diagnosis? Radiology 2003;226(1):47–52.

[19] Maki DD, Birnbaum BA, Chakraborty DP, et al. Renal cyst pseudoenhancement: beam-hardening effects on CT numbers. Radiology 1999;213(2):468–72.

[20] Abdulla C, Kalra MK, Saini S, et al. Pseudoenhancement of simulated renal cysts in a phantom using different multidetector CT scanners. AJR Am J Roentgenol 2002;179(6):1473–6.

[21] Bosniak MA. Difficulties in classifying cystic lesions of the kidney. Urol Radiol 1991;13(2):91–3.

[22] Israel GM, Bosniak MA. Follow-up CT of moderately complex cystic lesions of the kidney (Bosniak category IIF). AJR Am J Roentgenol 2003;181(3):627–33.

[23] Guinan P, Sobin LH, Algaba F, et al. TNM staging of renal cell carcinoma: Workgroup No. 3. Union International Contre le Cancer (UICC) and the American Joint Committee on Cancer (AJCC). Cancer 1997;80(5):992–3.

[24] Choyke PL, Walther MM, Wagner JR, et al. Renal cancer: preoperative evaluation with dual-phase three-dimensional MR angiography. Radiology 1997;205(3):767–71.

[25] Dunnick NR, Korobkin M. Imaging of adrenal incidentalomas: current status. AJR Am J Roentgenol 2002;179(3):559–68.

[26] Korobkin M, Giordano TJ, Brodeur FJ, et al. Adrenal adenomas: relationship between histologic lipid and CT and MR findings. Radiology 1996;200(3):743–7.

[27] Hood MN, Ho VB, Smirniotopoulos JG, et al. Chemical shift: the artifact and clinical tool revisited. Radiographics 1999;19(2):357–71.

[28] Israel GM, Korobkin M, Wang C, et al. Comparison of unenhanced CT and chemical shift MRI in evaluating lipid-rich adrenal adenomas. AJR Am J Roentgenol 2004;183(1):215–9.

[29] Elsayes KM, Narra VR, Leyendecker JR, et al. MRI of adrenal and extraadrenal pheochromocytoma. AJR Am J Roentgenol 2005;184(3):860–7.

[30] Kawashima A, Glockner JF, King BF Jr. CT urography and MR urography. Radiol Clin North Am 2003;41(5):945–61.

[31] Nolte-Ernsting CC, Staatz G, Tacke J, et al. MR urography today. Abdom Imaging 2003;28(2):191–209.

[32] Tekes A, Kamel I, Imam K, et al. Dynamic MRI of bladder cancer: evaluation of staging accuracy. AJR Am J Roentgenol 2005;184(1):121–7.

[33] Claus FG, Hricak H, Hattery RR. Pretreatment evaluation of prostate cancer: role of MR imaging and 1H MR spectroscopy. Radiographics 2004;24(Suppl 1):S167–80.

[34] Rajesh A, Coakley FV. MR imaging and MR spectroscopic imaging of prostate cancer. Magn Reson Imaging Clin N Am 2004;12(3):557–79; vii.

ELSEVIER
SAUNDERS

Urol Clin N Am 33 (2006) 319–328

UROLOGIC
CLINICS
of North America

Radionuclide Imaging in Urology

C. Richard Goldfarb, MD[a],*, Neil C. Srivastava, MD[a],
Aaron B. Grotas, MD[b], Fukiat Ongseng, MD[a],
Harris M. Nagler, MD[b]

[a]Department of Radiology, Beth Israel Medical Center, First Avenue at 16th Street, New York, NY 10003, USA
[b]Department of Urology, Beth Israel Medical Center, First Avenue at 16th Street, New York, NY 10003, USA

Radiopharmaceutics used in genitourinary imaging

Its unique sensitivity to functional changes makes renal scintigraphy with renography the imaging procedure of choice in the evaluation of conditions that induce focal alterations in kidney function or drainage. Because intravenous contrast is not used, scintigraphy neither damages the kidneys nor induces allergic reaction, and thus offers a clear advantage over intravenous pyelography (IVP) and CT. Additionally, it is better than IVP in visualizing both renal parenchyma and the collecting system in patients who have renal insufficiency or renal failure. Decisions regarding further work-up, type of treatment, duration of therapy, follow-up visits, and prognosis can be influenced by scintigraphy. In comparison with other diagnostic imaging modalities, nuclear medicine studies are noninvasive, with minimal patient discomfort, and no risk. Nuclear medicine studies are relatively nonoperator dependent and generally cost effective. They frequently provide unique functional information unavailable from ultrasound, IVP, CT, or MRI.

There are multiple radiopharmaceutic agents. Each agent has unique characteristics that allow it to provide the clinician with specific information. Therefore, it is important that the practitioner understand the radiopharmaceutic and its attributes, so that the appropriate study is ordered and the desired information provided.

Technetium^{99m}-diethylene triamine penta-acetic acid

Technetium^{99m}-diethylene triamine penta-acetic acid (^{99m}Tc-DTPA), is a chelating agent that has been in use since the 1970s. ^{99m}Tc-DTPA reaches equilibrium in the bloodstream approximately 1 to 2 hours after intravenous administration. It is lipid insoluble and therefore does not enter the cell. The portion that is not protein bound (roughly 90%–99%) is almost entirely removed from circulation by glomerular filtration. Therefore, it is the imaging agent most suited to measurement of glomerular filtration rate (GFR) [1]. ^{99m}Tc-DTPA is readily available, easy to prepare, and inexpensive. Early images using ^{99m}Tc-DTPA provide information about renal perfusion, whereas delayed images provide information about GFR (renal function) and the collecting system. A disadvantage of using DTPA is a small but variable degree of plasma protein binding, roughly 1% to 10%, which can result in an underestimation of the actual GFR. Because DTPA is almost exclusively filtered, adequate imaging of the collecting systems is GFR-dependent.

^{123}I or ^{131}I Hippuran

Hippuran, or ortho-iodohippuric acid, is an organic anion. The kidney secretes it so rapidly by way of glomerular filtration and tubular secretion that there is virtually none remaining in the renal arterial plasma after a single pass through the kidney. This attribute allows its clearance to be used as an estimation of effective renal plasma flow (ERPF). The major disadvantages of using

* Corresponding author.
E-mail address: rgoldfar@chpnet.org (C.R. Goldfarb).

0094-0143/06/$ - see front matter © 2006 Elsevier Inc. All rights reserved.
doi:10.1016/j.ucl.2006.03.006

hippuran are the radioisotopes used to label it. [131]I is a beta-emitter, which results in a high radiation dose per imageable photon. Moreover, the emitted photon is poorly imaged by conventional gamma cameras, owing to its high energy (364 kiloelectron volts (keV)). [123]I is much more suitable for imaging, with an emission of 159 keV, but it requires a cyclotron for production and has a short half-life of 13 hours. These factors, and its high expense, limit its use at most major medical centers.

Technetium[99m]-mercaptoacetyl triglycine

Technetium[99m]-mercaptoacetyl triglycine (^{99m}Tc-MAG3), has replaced hippuran for renal imaging at most facilities [2]. Like hippuran, it is cleared predominantly by tubular secretion. Unlike hippuran, it is labeled with ^{99m}Tc, an ideal agent for imaging because of its photon emission energy (140 keV), adequate half-life (6 hours), ease of preparation, and manageable expense. MAG3 is excreted predominantly by way of tubular secretion; however, extrarenal mechanisms account for 10% of the total clearance (mostly hepatobiliary). Because of its variable and slightly higher extrarenal clearance, MAG3 is less suitable than hippuran for estimating ERPF. ^{99m}Tc-MAG3 is extensively protein bound in plasma, substantially restricting its glomerular filtration and limiting its ability to measure GFR. The active secretion of MAG3, independent of GFR, makes it the agent of choice for imaging patients who have renal insufficiency or urinary obstruction.

Technetium[99m]-dimercaptosuccinic acid

Technetium [99m]-dimercaptosuccinic acid (^{99m}Tc-DMSA), is another chelating agent that has been adapted for use in renal imaging [3]. Tc-labeled DMSA localizes in the renal cortex, with negligible accumulation in the renal papilla and medulla. DMSA is therefore the radiopharmaceutic of choice for identifying cortical defects, locating aberrant kidneys, and, most importantly, for distinguishing benign-functioning space-occupying lesions, which typically are DMSA avid, from pathologic renal masses that appear as defects. Inability to image the collecting system and provide information on ureteral emptying is an obvious limitation of DMSA. In addition, renal tubular acidosis, certain medications, and tubulopathies have been shown to reduce renal DMSA uptake. Nevertheless, DMSA plays an important role in imaging renal cortical abnormalities.

Technetium[99m]-glucoheptonate

Technetium[99m]-glucoheptonate (^{99m}Tc-GHA), like DTPA, has been used in renal imaging for nearly 30 years [4]. Roughly one half of the activity in plasma is protein bound, and GHA is excreted partially by tubular secretion. Unlike other secreted agents, however, there is significant uptake of GHA in the renal cortex. GHA therefore has intermediate characteristics between tubularly secreted tracers (such as MAG3 and hippuran) and "cortical" tracers (DMSA). It is able to image both the cortex and the collecting systems. Unlike DMSA, abnormalities of acid-base balance have no effect on renal uptake. These characteristics can be an advantage, depending on the specific situation.

Role of nuclear medicine in upper urinary tract obstruction

Nuclear medicine plays a pivotal role in the evaluation of urinary tract obstruction. Although other imaging modalities (such as CT, ultrasound, and intravenous urography) display anatomic detail, only nuclear imaging can provide non-invasive information regarding dynamic function [5]. The unique information provided by nuclear medicine studies, including differential function between right and left, and clearance time, may be critical in patient management.

The radiopharmaceutic of choice in the setting of obstructive uropathy is ^{99m}Tc-MAG3, and the classic study performed is diuresis renography. A standardized protocol for this type of examination has been introduced [6]. Patients should be well hydrated before arrival. The study can be performed with the patient sitting up or lying supine. Flexibility of positioning and lack of dietary restriction provide distinct advantages over other imaging studies. The bladder is emptied immediately before starting the examination. Images of the kidneys and bladder are obtained for approximately 20 to 40 minutes after injection of the radiopharmaceutic. If an abnormal result is encountered, a diuretic (usually furosemide 0.5 mg/kg) is administered intravenously and additional images are obtained for another 15 to 20 minutes. Data analysis is performed by defining regions of interest over the kidneys and bladder, and a background area for comparison. The number of counts occurring in each region of interest, correcting for the background count, is then plotted over time. The resultant curves characterize the renogram.

The normal renogram curve has three distinct phases (Fig. 1). The first phase is characterized by a rapid rise immediately after radiopharmaceutic injection, reflecting the perfusion to the kidneys. The second phase of the renogram is characterized by a more gradual increase in counts over time, reflecting the renal clearance of the radiotracer. The normal curve peaks after 2 to 5 minutes, marking the beginning of the third phase of the renogram. This excretion phase is characterized by a gradual decline in renal counts over time, with a corresponding slow increase in bladder counts. The third phase, therefore, reflects the efficiency of urinary radiotracer excretion. The normal time required for one half of the tracer to leave the collecting system, or "half-time," is less than 10 minutes.

Renal function is evaluated primarily by the second phase of the renogram, when activity in each kidney is proportional to ERPF and, to a much lesser extent, GFR. Urinary obstruction, depending on its degree and duration, will often depress the slope of the second phase, altering the relative function assessment.

A normal renogram excludes clinically significant obstruction. When obstruction is present, the third phase of the renogram will be flattened to an extent dependent on its severity (Fig. 2). As obstruction becomes more severe or protracted, renal function is depressed and uptake is reduced (thus altering the second phase, as described earlier). When severe obstruction is present, uptake in the kidneys may be little more than the background count, resulting in nonvisualization of the affected urinary components.

A common cause of a false-positive "obstructive" renogram is slow elimination of the

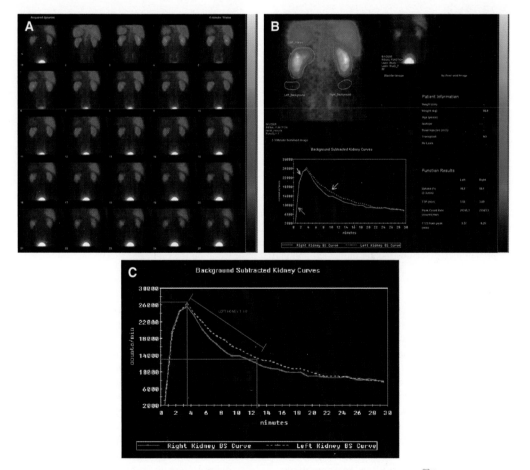

Fig. 1. Normal renogram. (*A*) Posterior planar images obtained at 1-minute intervals following ^{99m}Tc-MAG3 injection. (*B*) Note the three distinct phases of the renogram curves (*red, blue, and yellow arrows denoting phases 1, 2, and 3, respectively*) and emptying half-times of less than 10 minutes. (*C*) How the emptying half-time is measured.

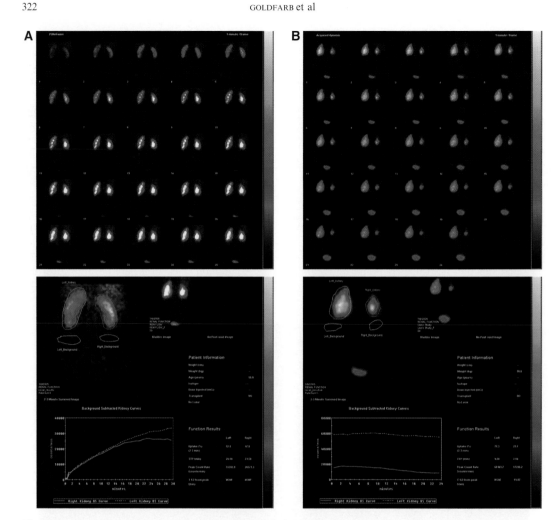

Fig. 2. Total left-sided obstruction with partial right-sided obstruction. Posterior planar images of a 58-year-old woman with a history of prior left ureteropelvic junction obstruction. (*A*) Note delayed excretion in both kidneys. (*B*) Following the administration of furosemide, there is no response in the left kidney and suboptimal response in the right. These findings represent high-grade obstruction on the left and partial obstruction on the right. BS, background subtracted.

radiotracer due to urinary stasis. This potentially confounding factor is overcome by the routine administration of a diuretic during the course of the examination to induce a high urinary flow rate. This procedure is referred to as a diuretic renal scan. A nonobstructed urinary system will respond to the administration of the diuretic with an abrupt decline in renal activity (Fig. 3). A more gradual decline in activity after diuretic administration reflects a "suboptimal" response, and is interpreted as equivalent to obstruction. Other potential sources of false-positive renograms are unrecognized dehydration (which often produces a suboptimal response to diuretic); poor renal

function; and massive dilatation of the collecting system with urinary stasis that is not the result of obstruction. A full or nearly full bladder will physiologically impair renal washout; therefore, it is best to keep the bladder relatively decompressed throughout the study.

Another possible pattern of the renogram curve in response to diuretic administration is the "delayed decompensation" pattern. Initial response to diuretic administration is good, but at a certain point the curve flattens out or begins to rise, reflecting increased flow rates that partially obstructed systems cannot tolerate. These systems begin to decompensate, resulting in further

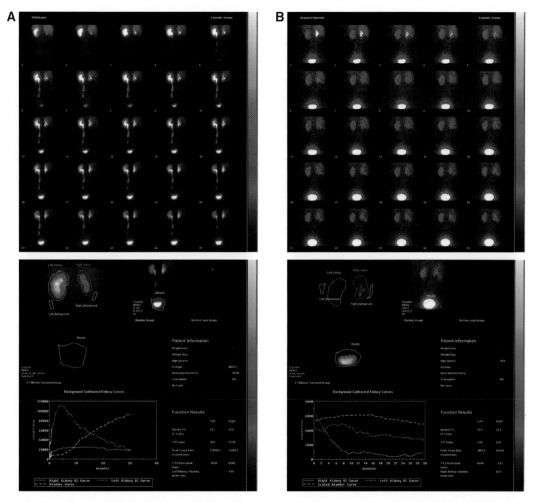

Fig. 3. Nonobstructive hydronephrosis. A 70-year-old man with a history of colon cancer and hydronephrosis. Apparent poor excretion from the right kidney (*A*) demonstrates good response to the administration of furosemide, indicating nonobstructive hydronephrosis (*B*). BS, background subtracted.

dilatation. The goal of diuresis renography is to determine the urodynamic significance of a dilated collecting system. This information is crucial for proper patient management.

Medical renal disease

The differential diagnosis of acute renal failure includes urinary tract obstruction and primary medical renal disease, such as acute tubular necrosis (ATN), interstitial nephritis, and glomerulonephritis. Often, medical renal diseases can be diagnosed and differentiated using radionuclide assays. As originally described in the renal transplant literature, the ^{99m}Tc-MAG3 renal scan can also differentiate among ATN obstruction, and other medical renal diseases [7].

Blaustein and colleagues [8] have suggested a distinct pattern of ATN in MAG3 renal imaging in native kidneys. They reported preserved renal perfusion with gradually increasing parenchymal uptake for 60 minutes, with minimal or no excretion into the upper urinary tract. Unlike patients who have ATN, patients who have glomerulonephritis or interstitial nephritis demonstrate poor renal uptake of tracer, and a renal biopsy may be required to make a diagnosis. Renal scans have also been used to diagnose renal transplant rejection. These scans show impaired kidney perfusion and poor parenchymal uptake of tracer [9].

Nuclear medicine in renal infection imaging

Radionuclide imaging can be used to identify and monitor infections encountered in urologic practice. [67]Gallium citrate and [111]indium- or ^{99m}Tc-labeled autologous white blood cells concentrate in inflamed and infected tissues. No currently available tracers can distinguish infection from sterile inflammation. Gallium also accumulates in some tumors and cannot distinguish between benign and malignant inflammatory processes. [67]Gallium-citrate is injected intravenously and imaging of the abdomen is commenced 48 hours later. A repeat study can be obtained at 72 hours to differentiate suspected inflammatory or neoplastic lesions from physiologic gallium accumulation in the bowel. If there is clinical urgency to make a diagnosis earlier, imaging at 24 hours or even at 4 to 6 hours will often identify a focus of infection, although detail will be suboptimal before 2 days. Also, physiologic uptake of gallium in the kidneys can persist up to 24 hours after injection and can obscure renal infection. A renal scan or colloid liver/spleen scan may be obtained in the same position as the gallium scan, for subtraction, to localize any abnormal sites of uptake more accurately. Recently, single photon emission tomography (SPECT) fused with CT has markedly improved lesion localization.

[111]Indium or ^{99m}Tc white cell imaging requires drawing approximately 60 mL of blood, followed by labeling with tracer, and reinjection. Imaging with [111]indium WBC commences at 24 hours, whereas ^{99m}Tc WBC are imaged several hours after labeling and reinjection. Neither tracer is ideal for urologic imaging because of physiologic accumulation in the kidneys and bladder, a problem not encountered with gallium as long as images are obtained more than 24 hours after injection.

Acute pyelonephritis

Renal cortical scintigraphy with ^{99m}Tc-DMSA or ^{99m}Tc-GHA can detect acute pyelonephritis and areas of scarring in chronic pyelonephritis. It can demonstrate focal or global areas of decreased uptake of tracer with preservation of the renal contour. Corresponding cortical abnormalities are present in 50% to 90% of children with febrile UTI [10]. In acute pyelonephritis, scintigraphy shows focal areas of decreased activity or focal defects, whereas other imaging modalities may be normal or show minor anatomic changes. Scars may be the end result of reflux or infection of the renal parenchyma as in acute pyelonephritis.

Chronic pyelonephritis

Renal scintigraphy is the procedure of choice for long-term follow-up of the functional and anatomic status of the kidneys in patients who have chronic pyelonephritis. Although parenchymal or drainage system anatomy may show little change and be difficult to evaluate, scintigraphy can determine quantitatively whether the disease is stable, progressive, or resolving.

Renal abscesses

Renal abscesses usually result from ascending spread of urinary tract pathogens. Clinical presentation is usually symptomatic, with fever and flank pain similar to that of pyelonephritis, but a significant number of patients may have negative urinalysis when the abscess fails to communicate with the collecting system. Although scintigraphy may show the abscess as a focal defect, the image is not diagnostic. Gallium or WBC imaging may be capable of localizing the area of abscess, yet in most circumstances differentiation from pyelonephritis is difficult. Gallium and labeled white cells have been useful occasionally in the detection of abdominal abscesses, most notably those involving the psoas muscle.

New radiopharmaceutics for diagnosis of inflammatory conditions

Fanolesomab (FNB), a ^{99m}Tc-labeled murine anti-CD 15 IgM monoclonal antibody that specifically targets neutrophils, is a novel radiopharmaceutic designed to detect and localize infections. FNB has shown promise in detecting infectious states, such as appendicitis or other intra-abdominal infection. FNB has the advantage of imaging within minutes of injection, having a ^{99m}Tc label (allowing better count rate and image detail), and ease and speed of preparation. FNB is likely to replace gallium and labeled white cells for scinitgraphic infection detection, except in the kidneys, where physiologic uptake limits FNB's accuracy.

Nuclear medicine in oncological imaging

Nuclear medicine imaging for the management of urologic malignancy has expanded beyond its early role as a test for metastatic bone disease.

Metastatic disease

Conventional radionuclide imaging has a long history in the investigation of bone metastases in urologic malignancies. Skeletal scintigraphy (radionuclide bone scan) is the most sensitive method for detecting bone metastases (Fig. 4) [11]. False-negative results in patients undergoing metastatic evaluation for prostate cancer can occur, however, especially in the marrow-containing vertebra [12]. MRI is particularly sensitive for detecting lesions in this area. A positive bone scan is not specific for malignancy and often requires confirmation by plain radiography, CT, or MRI. A thorough history, including information regarding recent fractures, surgery, or known arthritic conditions, will reduce misinterpretation.

Patients who have diffuse metastatic bone involvement demonstrate uniformly increased uptake of radionuclide in the skeletal structures with either a faint or absent renogram. This phenomenon is referred to as a "superscan" because the exquisite skeletal detail is mistaken occasionally by inexperienced interpreters as a normal bone scan [13]. It can be seen in patients who have metastatic prostate cancer with diffuse bony metastases. For the osteoblastic bone metastases typically found in prostate cancer, conventional bone scan

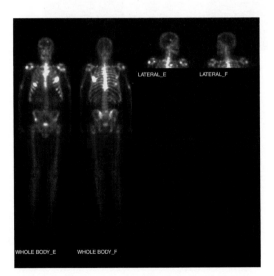

Fig. 4. Positive bone scan of a 54-year-old man with a history of metastatic prostate cancer. Multiple foci of metastatic disease are noted involving the skull, mandible, cervical spine, thoracic spine, ribs, manubrium, scapula, both humeri, the sacrum, the iliac bones, and both femurs.

appears to be superior to FDG-PET (positron emission tomography) [14].

In recent years, PET has been used increasingly in detecting, staging, and monitoring a wide variety of malignancies (Fig. 5). In urologic practice, FDG-PET can examine regional nodal status, disclose distant metastases, and discover local recurrence in prostate, bladder, and testicular cancers.

Prostate cancer

Although conventional ultrasonography or MRI is able to identify the anatomic features of prostate cancer, several studies have identified a niche for PET scan in investigating nodal involvement and detecting recurrence in the postoperative or postradiation field. There may be a role for PET in monitoring patients who have hormone refractory or metastatic prostate undergoing investigational and novel therapies.

Testicular cancer

Staging of testicular cancer includes histology, serum tumor markers, and CT. Although retroperitoneal nodes may not be enlarged by CT criteria, retroperitoneal lymph node dissection may reveal positive nodal disease in 20% to 30% of cases. Overall, CT has been reported to have false-negative rates exceeding 50% and false-positive rates as high as 40%. FDG-PET has been shown to be superior to CT in staging testicular cancer [15], but, as with a CT scan, the resolution of a PET scan limits its ability to detect small micrometastases. Theoretically, PET may provide a tool to differentiate fibrosis and necrosis from persistent or recurrent active disease. In addition, PET may be useful in following patients' responses to chemotherapy [16].

Bladder cancer

Detection of bladder cancer using PET is limited because FDG is excreted physiologically into the urinary tract. Nevertheless, some small studies have reported the usefulness of FDG-PET for the evaluation of recurrent or residual disease. There may be a role also for detecting lymph node involvement. Further studies are necessary before a recommendation can be made about the use of PET in bladder cancer [17].

Pheochromocytoma

Pheochromocytomas arise from the chromaffin cells of the adrenal medulla. They can cause severe

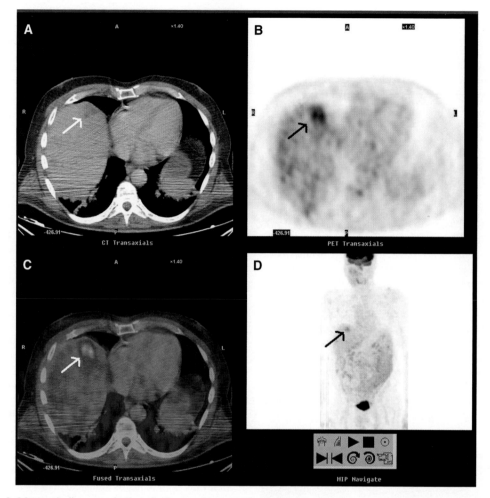

Fig. 5. Metastatic disease to the liver. A 63-year-old man with suspected renal cell carcinoma who underwent a PET-CT for metastatic work-up. CT (*A*), PET (*B*), PET-CT fusion (*C*), and whole-body PET images (*D*) demonstrate a hypermetabolic lesion in the dome of the liver likely representing metastatic disease (*arrows*).

hypertension, and therefore it is vitally important to diagnose and identify all sites harboring malignant cells. Metaiodobenzylguanidine (MIBG) scintigraphy, using ^{123}I or ^{131}I, is especially useful for the detection of ectopic pheochromocytomas and also for the identification of metastatic or locally recurrent disease because, unlike ultrasonography, CT, or MRI, it is a whole-body, functional imaging technique [18]. Pheochromocytomas are seen as focal areas of increased MIBG activity. The sensitivity of MIBG scintigraphy in detecting functioning pheochromocytomas is slightly less than 90% and its specificity exceeds 90% if correlated with CT or MRI.

Although, MIBG scan is the gold standard for detecting ectopic pheochromocytomas, a role for PET scan may be emerging. There have been several case reports of FDG-PET detecting ectopic active tumors in patients who had a false-negative MIBG scan [19]. If patients have biochemically proven pheochromocytoma, and CT, MRI, or MIBG fails to identify the source, FDG-PET may be useful for finding ectopic or metastatic disease.

Palliation of bone pain in cancer patients

A significant number of patients who have advanced cancer have moderate to severe bone pain. The current standard of therapy involves the use of narcotics; however, significant side effects and quality of life issues are associated with this type of treatment. A number of radiopharmaceutics are currently available for reduction of metastatic bone pain, and their use can diminish the need for narcotics and thus improve overall quality of life for patients who have advanced cancer [20].

Most of the data supporting the use of radiopharmaceutics for the treatment of bone pain come from studies on metastatic breast, prostate, and lung cancer, although any cancer that has a positive bone scan should be amenable to treatment [21]. The duration of response generally ranges from a few weeks to a few months, and thus treatments every few months are the typical standard. Currently, three radiopharmaceutics are commercially available for bone pain palliation: sodium phosphate (^{32}P), strontium-89 chloride (^{89}Sr), and samarium-153 (^{153}Sm).

Sodium phosphate

^{32}P has been in use since the 1950s to relieve bone pain from metastatic prostate and breast cancer. After intravenous or oral administration, radioactive phosphate is incorporated into hydroxyapatite. Early studies demonstrated good response rates, on the order of 60% to 85%, and more recent data have confirmed their efficacy [22]. Major advantages of ^{32}P include the ability to administer it orally, the fact that it does not have to be sterile or completely free of pyrogens, and its relatively low expense [23].

Strontium-89 chloride

^{89}Sr, like ^{32}P, has been used successfully for bone pain palliation for many years. A comprehensive review by Silberstein and colleagues [21] of 18 publications demonstrated an overall response rate of 65%, with the amount of response directly proportional to the administered dose.

Samarium-153-ethylene-diaminetetramethylenephosphonate

Samarium-153-ethylene-diaminetetramethylenephosphonate binds hydroxyapatite through chemisorption and a hydrolysis reaction with oxygen on the hydroxyapatite molecule. Several studies have shown response rates of 55% to 80%, with no additional effects demonstrated at higher doses [24].

The primary adverse reaction from these radiopharmaceutics is myelotoxicity, and severe cases resulting in fatalities using ^{89}Sr and ^{153}Sm have been described. These deaths were the result of severe thrombocytopenia, which may have a multifactorial etiology in patients who have advanced cancer. An initial 48 to 72 hour increase in pain, known as the "flare phenomenon," has also been described in up to two thirds of patients and has been associated with a therapeutic palliative response.

Summary

Urologists use radiotracers most frequently in the assessment of kidney function and the detection of postrenal obstruction. Nuclear medicine studies are also of value in the localization of abdominal infection, the differential diagnosis of renal transplant complications, and the staging of genitourinary malignancies. Recently, PET using 18F-flurodeoxyglucose has expanded the role of radionuclide imaging in oncology. Preliminary research has been done. However, the application of this technology to urologic malignancies may be limited. Currently, radiolabeled monoclonal antibodies and positron tracers are being evaluated for both diagnostic and therapeutic applications for urologic malignancies. Radiopharmaceutics are likely to occupy a significant but changing role in the urologic armamentarium.

References

[1] Klopper JF, Hauser W, Atkins HL. Evaluation of ^{99m}Tc-DTPA for the measurement of glomerular filtration rate. J Nucl Med 1972;13:107–10.

[2] Fritzberg AR, Kasina S, Eshima D. Synthesis and biological evaluation of Tc-99m MAG3 as a hippuran replacement. J Nucl Med 1986;27:111–6.

[3] Lin TH, Khentigan A, Winchell HS. A ^{99m}Tc chelate substitute for organomercurial renal agents. J Nucl Med 1974;15:34–5.

[4] Kahn PC, Dewanjee MK, Brown SS. Routine renal imaging after ^{99m}Tc-glucoheptonate brain scans. J Nucl Med 1976;17:786–7.

[5] Britton K, Nimmon CC, Whitfield HN, et al. Obstructive nephropathy: successful evaluation with radionuclides. Lancet 1979;1:905–7.

[6] Gambhir SS, Ell, PJ. Nuclear medicine in clinical diagnosis and treatment. London: Churchill-Livingstone; 2004.

[7] Lin E. Significance of early tubular extraction in the first minute of Tc-99m MAG3 renal transplant scintigraphy. Clin Nucl Med 1998;23(4):217.

[8] Blaustein D, et al. The role of Technetium-99m Mag3 renal imaging in the diagnosis of acute

tubular necrosis of native kidneys. Clin Nucl Med 2002;27(3):167.

[9] Dubovsky EV. Evaluation of renal transplants. In: Henkin RA, et al, editors. Nuclear medicine. St. Louis, MO: Mosby; 1996. p. 1097–109.

[10] Kawashima A. Radiologic evaluation of patients with renal infections. Infect Dis Clin North Am 2003;17:433–56.

[11] Narayan P, Lillian D, Hellstrom W, et al. The benefits of combining early radionuclide renal scintigraphy with routine bone scans in patients with prostate cancer. J Urol 1988;140:1448.

[12] Ball JD, Maynard CD. Nuclear imaging in urology. Urol Clin North Am 1979;6:321.

[13] Kim SE, Kim DY, Lee DS, et al. Absent or faint renal uptake on bone scan-etiology and significance in metastatic bone disease. Clin Nucl Med 1991;16:545.

[14] Hain S, Massey M. Positron emission tomography for urological tumors. BJU International 2003; 92(2):159–64.

[15] Hain SF, et al. Fluorodeoxyglucose positron emission tomography in the evaluation of germ cell tumours at relapse. Br J Cancer 2000;83(7):863–9.

[16] Mikhaeel N, et al. FDG-PET after two to three cycles of chemotherapy predicts progression-free and overall survival in high-grade non-Hodgkin lymphoma. Ann Oncol 2005;16(9):1514–23.

[17] Kumar R. PET in the management of urologic malignancies. Radiol Clin North Am 2004;42:1151.

[18] Genitourinary imaging: radionuclide imaging. In: Grainger RG, Allison D, Dixon AK, editors. Diagnostic radiology: a textbook of medical imaging. 4th edition. Churchill Livingstone, Inc; 2001.

[19] Ezuddin S, Fragkaki C. MIBG and FDG PET findings in a patient with malignant pheochromocytoma: a significant discrepancy. Clin Nucl Med 2005;30(8):579.

[20] Atkins HL, Srivastava SC. Radiopharmaceutics for bone malignancy therapy. J Nucl Med Technol 1998;26:80–3.

[21] Silberstein E. Bone cancer therapy. In: Nuclear medicine: oncology. Society of Nuclear Medicine; 2004. p. 261–75.

[22] Silberstein EB. The treatment of painful osseous metastases with phosphorus-32-labeled phosphates. Semin Oncol 1993;20(Suppl 2):10–21.

[23] Nair N. Relative efficacy of ^{32}P and ^{89}Sr in palliation in skeletal metastases. J Nucl Med 1999;40: 256–61.

[24] Resche I, Chatal JF, Pecking A, et al. A dose-controlled study of ^{153}Sm-ethylene-diaminetetra-methylenephosphonate (EDTMP) in the treatment of patients with painful bone metastases. Eur J Cancer 1997;33:1583–91.

ELSEVIER
SAUNDERS

Urol Clin N Am 33 (2006) 329–337

UROLOGIC
CLINICS
of North America

Newer Modalities of Ultrasound Imaging and Treatment of the Prostate

Gilad E. Amiel, MD, Kevin M. Slawin, MD*

*Baylor Prostate Center, Scott Department of Urology, Baylor College of Medicine,
6560 Fannin, Suite 2100, Houston, TX 77030, USA*

In the past decade, a wide array of imaging modalities has been studied in an attempt to better image the prostate gland. Most of this effort was directed toward evaluating modalities to assess tumor in the prostate. However, significant improvement has been made in the evaluation of benign prostatic hypertrophy (BPH) and bladder outlet obstruction (BOO).

Imaging of the prostate in BPH is focused on assessing prostate size to best evaluate treatment for BPH and to exclude the presence of prostate cancer. Although there is continuous clinical research on the appropriate evaluation of BPH, the American Urological Association (AUA) and the International Consultation on BPH do not currently recommend imaging of the prostate gland as a routine. Nonetheless, gray scale transabdominal and transrectal ultrasound (TRUS), have been extensively evaluated for the assessment of BPH. Specifically, TRUS has been shown to reliably assess anatomical size, prostatic texture, and volume of the transitional zone. Transabdominal ultrasound is less invasive and is mainly used to assess bladder residual volume and the upper tracts.

For the evaluation of patients with prostate cancer, ultrasound and computed tomography (CT) have become the standard. Conventional ultrasound is not sufficiently sensitive or specific to detect prostate cancer [1]. TRUS serves to guide prostate biopsies, but is not reliable for staging, which commonly is being done by CT or magnetic resonance imaging (MRI), which has been available since 1984. Although CT and MRI have a high sensitivity for detecting lymph node metastases, their sensitivity for local disease is limited [2], and despite being the most accurate imaging techniques available for assessment of the prostate, they are expensive and have limited availability. Additionally, a large variation in reported staging accuracy has been documented [3,4]. These inconsistencies are related to variations in technique, sample size, and study population, and the ever-changing state-of-the-art technology. We will review the gray-scale ultrasound techniques currently available for the assessment of the prostate gland, and then focus on the new ultrasound imaging technologies for evaluating benign and malignant disease in the prostate, including their degree of acceptance as reported in the literature.

Conventional sonographic evaluation of the prostate

Transrectal ultrasound (TRUS) is an effective technique for calculating the volume of the prostate gland. Hendrikx and colleagues [5] compared ultrasonic prostatic volumes with physical measurements of completely removed specimens from human cadavers, and demonstrated a high correlation between the two measurements. Several methods for the sonographic measurement of prostatic volume have been established. In planimetric volumetry, the volume is calculated from the sum of cross-sectional areas of the prostate, and is considered the most accurate method of measuring the volume of the prostate [6,7]. However, this method is considered time-consuming

* Corresponding author.
E-mail address: kslawin@bcm.tmc.edu
(K.M. Slawin).

and tedious. Alternatively, using a formula describing the prostate as a spheroid structure, and using half the mean of width, height, and length as radius, one can calculate prostatic volume with reasonable accuracy.

Over the past decade, conventional gray-scale TRUS has revolutionized the early detection and management of prostatic disease, in particular prostate cancer. TRUS was found to be invaluable for accurately mapping and systematically taking biopsies of the prostate gland. However, as a screening tool for prostate cancer its sensitivity and specificity are low when compared with those for other diagnostic tools such as the serum prostate-specific antigen (PSA), percent free PSA, and digital rectal examination (DRE). TRUS is highly operator dependent, and data on the accuracy of ultrasound for staging has been inconsistent. Salo and colleagues [8] in 1987 reported a sensitivity of 86%, specificity of 94%, positive predictive value of 92%, and negative predictive value of 89% for predicting extracapsular invasion. Shortly thereafter, additional reports showed less favorable results of TRUS being able to accurately predict extracapsular invasion, with sensitivity between 23% and 66%, specificity between 46% and 86%, positive predictive value between 50% and 62%, and negative predictive value between 49% and 69% [9–12]. Augustin and coworkers [13] have recently reported that TRUS-visible lesions are found in more than 50% of patients with nonpalpable prostatic lesions, and that these tumors demonstrate significantly worse pathological stages and larger volumes than lesions that are also not visible by TRUS ($P = .002$). It has been well documented, that the majority of tumors have a hypoechoic echogenic pattern, although isoechoic or hyperechoic lesions may contain cancerous tissues as well [14]. A significant correlation between Gleason score and echogenicity has been found, with the majority of hypoechoic tumors being moderately or poorly differentiated and isoechoic lesions well or moderately differentiated [14]. These findings imply that tumors detected by ultrasound in many cases can be clinically important, and should not be interpreted as latent or incidental carcinomas. Since other abnormalities of the prostate can also produce hypoechoic changes, it may be difficult to differentiate prostatitis, infarction, and atrophy from prostate carcinoma. Nonetheless, because of the tendency of prostate cancer to develop in the peripheral zone, a hypoechoic lesion in the prostatic capsule is more suspicious than a similar lesion in the transitional zone, which is most commonly BPH. Additionally, any region that is abnormal during digital rectal examination should be carefully investigated. In many cases, ultrasound can underestimate the actual size of a tumor [15], with an average underestimate of 4.8 mm in diameter compared with histopathologic whole-mount sections [14]. Based on these findings, TRUS cannot stand alone as a useful tool for predicting cancer volume or for making treatment decisions. However, for follow-up purposes, TRUS can adequately demonstrate volume decrease and size reduction of hypoechoic lesions after initiation of androgen deprivation therapy [16,17].

Newer modalities

Color and power Doppler

To improve the ability of sonography to detect and correctly characterize lesions, a wide array of new technologies has been assessed over the past few years. Color Doppler has been employed with a rationale to identify blood vessels within the tumor. Standard color Doppler and power Doppler allow investigation of normal and abnormal blood flow in the prostate. Blood vessels within tumors tend to demonstrate low impedance or resistance to flow. This phenomenon has been shown previously by color and pulsed Doppler in cancers of the breast, liver, kidney, and ovary. In prostate cancer, increased flow has been identified in this abnormal tumor vasculature. Several studies have investigated whether color Doppler can improve the sensitivity and specificity of conventional gray-scale TRUS in detecting early stages of prostate cancer. Early studies using color Doppler characterized the normal vascular anatomy of the prostate [18,19]. Subsequently, the clinical utility of color Doppler in the assessment of altered patterns of blood flow as seen in prostatic disease has been evaluated by several investigators. Some studies showed that color Doppler did not add significant information to gray-scale TRUS in detecting early stages of prostate cancer [20,21]. Others demonstrated varying degrees of benefit [22,23]. Overall, the sensitivity of color Doppler for the diagnosis of prostate cancer ranged between 49% and 87%, and specificity ranged between 38% and 93% [20–22,24,25]. Color Doppler has an excellent positive predictive value for tumor detection, compared with gray-scale TRUS or MR imaging, although it provides a lower sensitivity rate [26]. Nonetheless, a substantial number of cancers are not detected even by means of high-frequency Doppler ultrasound [26].

Power Doppler is considered the next generation of color Doppler imaging. Depending on the amplitude of the signal, the image is displayed with varying hue and brightness. The total energy of the Doppler signal is displayed by color [27]. Power Doppler relies on the amplitude of the signal to determine the density of the red blood cells, regardless of their direction or velocity of flow. This is contrary to conventional color Doppler, which uses a method of calculating the mean frequency shift of the signal to verify the velocity and direction of flow of red blood cells. Power Doppler has the advantage of increased sensitivity for detecting small, low-flow blood vessels [28]. This increased sensitivity of the power Doppler allows for more accurate visualization of blood flow within the prostate, and adds to the value of power Doppler TRUS as a diagnostic tool. Since power and color Dopplers are currently available on transrectal probes, the diagnosis of BPH can be improved by the assessment of intraprostatic vascularity [29–31]. Power Doppler imaging is considered to be 3 to 5 times more sensitive for the assessment of blood flow than color Doppler imaging [31]. It is superior because of a lack of aliasing, little angle dependence, and low noise background.

Both benign and malignant disease may distort the normal blood flow patterns in the prostate. Therefore, it is important to understand the vascular anatomy of the normal prostate as presented via power Doppler imaging. Leventis and colleagues [32] studied the blood flow patterns within the various zones of the prostate and correlated these findings with the zonal anatomy of the prostate as depicted by gray-scale TRUS. They managed to visualize separate branches of the capsular vessels that distributed radially into the peripheral and central zones, and then come together toward the center of the gland. Urethral vessels were observed in the transition zone coursing from the bladder neck to the verumontanum (Fig. 1). The neurovascular bundles were seen to lie posterolaterally along the longitudinal axis of the gland. The resistive index (RI) of the blood vessels in the urethra and the capsular vessels was fairly similar. However, the RI of the neurovascular bundles and that of the prostatic vessels were significantly different ($P < .001$). Leventis and colleagues also demonstrated that the vascular anatomy of the normal prostate can be

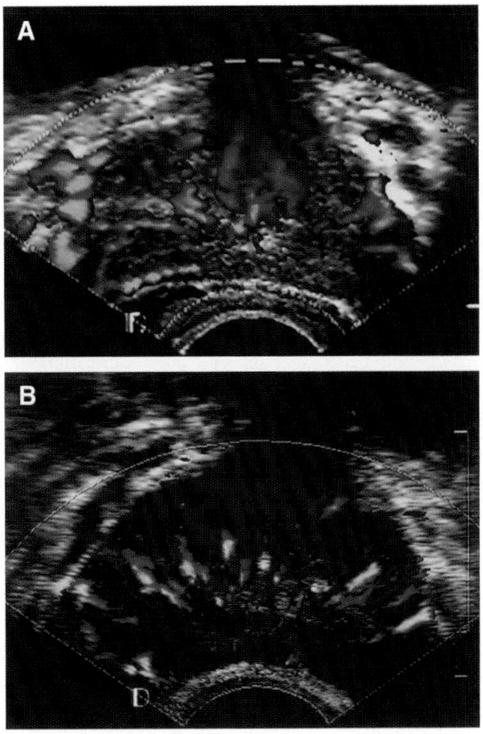

Fig. 1. Power Doppler imaging of the prostate: mid-prostate level, in axial scanning. (A) The capsular vessels are visualized entering and distributed in the boundaries of the peripheral zone, as urethral vessels are visualized en route along the urethra. (B) This topographic image displays the symmetric distribution of the capsular vessels within the peripheral zone. There is a hypovascular appearance of the anterior fibromuscular stroma and of the posterior mid-segment of the gland.

displayed by power Doppler, which is superior to color Doppler. This led to the systematic assessment of the vascular anatomy of BPH and prostate cancer.

Power Doppler ultrasonography of the prostate has clearly demonstrated that the RI increases significantly in BPH [29–31]. Tsuru and coworkers [33] measured the RI before and after transurethral vaporization of the prostate in a group of BPH patients to investigate the changes of RI after surgery and its correlation to improvement of lower urinary tract symptoms (LUTS). They assessed 43 patients, in a series of tests before and 1, 3, and 6 months after surgery, with a mean follow-up of 9.1 months. All evaluated parameters, including the International Prostate Symptom Scores (IPSS), quality of life scores, post-voiding residual urine volumes (PVR), and maximum urinary flow rates (Qmax) that were evaluated, were correlated with changes in total prostatic volume (TPV) and RI as measured by power Doppler. The investigators have found that all of these parameters significantly improved and that they all correlated with the reduced RI after surgery. Interestingly, the change in RI was observed last, after all the other parameters had improved. The authors suggested that RI can serve to measure the severity of BPH and the degree of pressure within the prostate.

It is widely accepted that tumors enhance neovascularization. This has been demonstrated in a variety of cancers, including prostate cancer [34–37]. In the prostate, it has been shown that increased vascularity can be found in hypoechoic gray-scale lesions, and that this is correlated with an increased likelihood of prostate cancer [21,22,38]. These measurements were largely based on an attempt to quantify the overall number of blood vessels in the prostate and not on vascular density, which measures the number of vessels per unit area of the tissue. However, current pathologic literature that links angiogenesis to cancer uses the measurement of vascular density as an estimate of vascular activity [36,39,40].

Early studies using Doppler sonography and power Doppler techniques demonstrated that hypervascularity correlates with increased Gleason score. Cornud and colleagues [41] prospectively evaluated 94 patients with color Doppler before undergoing radical prostatectomy. They found that the evaluation of hypoechoic lesions at the time of biopsy with these two modalities is useful in predicting increased Gleason score and the aggressiveness of the tumor. However, later studies trying to confirm the added value of color and power Doppler were disappointing.

Early studies of Doppler ultrasound of the prostate involved the use of Doppler frequencies in the range of 5–7.5 MHz. However, later studies demonstrated superior Doppler detection of blood flow within the prostate with a probe incorporating a frequency of 9 MHz [42]. Halpern and colleagues [26] compared the detection of cancer with targeted biopsies performed on the basis of the results of color and power Doppler examination at 9 MHz using a systematic sextant biopsy approach. They evaluated 62 patients with transrectal gray-scale, color, and power Doppler ultrasound. After obtaining up to four targeted biopsies based on Doppler findings from each patient, they performed a modified sextant biopsy. The yields of each method were compared.

Eighteen (29%) of the 62 patients had cancer. In 11 patients, cancer was detected with both sextant and targeted biopsies; in 6 patients it was detected with only sextant biopsies, and in 1 it was detected only with targeted biopsies. The positive biopsy rate for targeted biopsies was 13% (24 of 185 cores). This was insignificantly higher than the 9.7% for sextant biopsies (36 of 372 cores; $P = .1$). Interestingly, the overall identification of positive sextant biopsy sites was close to random chance for all imaging modalities (gray-scale area under the curve, 0.53; color Doppler, 0.50 and power Doppler, 0.47). The authors concluded that high-frequency color or power Doppler is not reliable for detecting cancerous lesions in the prostate gland, and that these methods would probably miss a significant number of cancers that would be detected with sextant biopsy. These disappointing results were verified by other groups as well [43].

Arger and colleagues [44], in an attempt to improve the clinical efficacy of these new technologies, compared two methods that quantitatively assess the vascularity of the prostate using Doppler imaging. Total vascularity counts the overall number of blood vessels over a predetermined imaged area. Vascular density measures the fraction of the mean area occupied by blood vessels in multiple cross-sections of the prostate. The authors wanted to study the differences between these two measurements of vascularity in the prostate, and whether they could correlate them to pathologic diagnosis. They also evaluated the relationship between hypoechoic areas, hypervascularity, and pathologic diagnosis. When 90 patients underwent biopsy, patients eventually diagnosed with BPH, PIN, and prostate cancer did not demonstrate a substantial difference in vascularity by either total vascularity or vascular density. Interestingly, only in BPH was the total vascular volume in the central gland significantly higher than in the peripheral parts of the gland. However, the vascular density in the peripheral gland was 2.5 times higher than in the central gland. Of 31 focal hypoechoic lesions, 71% were hypervascular, but only 23% were diagnosed with tumor. The authors concluded that although quantitative analysis based on vascular density, which is more comparable with histopathologic findings, demonstrated that the peripheral gland is more vascular than the central gland, the overall pathologic categories were not separable by the tested vascular measurements. All pathologic categories expressed low, moderate, or high vascularity, and, therefore, vascular areas by definition cannot distinguish between benign or malignant tissue or add to the diagnostic value of focal hypoechoic areas in the prostate. These recent findings supported previous reports that hypervascularity is not an independent factor in distinguishing between various pathologic entities, and therefore cannot serve as a tool to decrease the number of prostate biopsies (Fig. 2).

Three-dimensional ultrasound of the prostate

Three-dimensional (3D) ultrasound was developed as a noninvasive method to generate whole volume images of solid structures. Early studies on prostate imaging identified several advantages of this method over 2D imaging [45]. This is because conventional TRUS uses two dimensions to visualize a 3D disease process. Currently, 3D TRUS systems are available for prostate imaging. These machines process a series of sequentially overlaid images, resulting in a single image of higher resolution and quality (Fig. 3). However, the image acquired using a standard gray-scale 3D endorectal transducer is similar to the conventional 2D TRUS. Therefore, no advantage could be found in the diagnosis of prostate cancer. This is because up to 80% of hypoechoic lesions diagnosed by TRUS are not cancerous [46], and 50% of nonpalpable tumors larger than 1 cm are not visualized by ultrasound [47].

Hamper and colleagues [48] evaluated gray-scale 3D TRUS in 16 men before prostate biopsy. 3D coronally reconstructed images were superior to 2D TRUS in identifying tumors and extra-glandular disease. Garg and colleagues [49] performed 3D TRUS using a conventional gray-scale scanner in 36 newly diagnosed clinically localized prostate

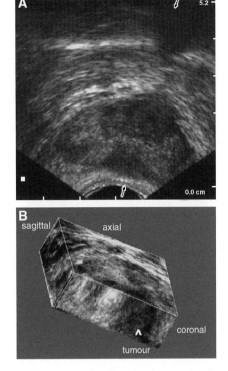

Fig. 3. 3D power color Doppler sonography demonstrating a malignant lesion in the right peripheral zone. (*A*) Conventional 2D gray-scale image. (*B*) Three-dimensional image.

cancer patients. The 3D imaging demonstrated a 94% overall staging accuracy, 80% sensitivity, and 96% specificity. Staging accuracy compared with that with 2D TRUS was significantly improved (94% versus 72%, *P* < .05). Strasser

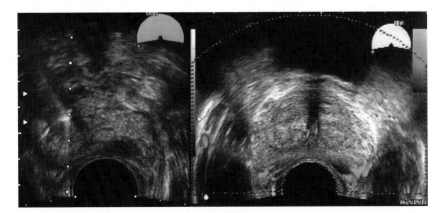

Fig. 2. (*A*) Gray-scale trans-rectal ultrasound demonstrating a hypoechoic lesion that was diagnosed as Gleason Grade 4 cancer of the prostate. (*B*) The same lesion as seen in power Doppler.

and colleagues [50] investigated 107 men before radical prostatectomy. Three-dimensional TRUS demonstrated 87% sensitivity, 94% specificity, and a 97% Positive Predictive Value (PPV) for extracapsular extension. Of 16 men with histologically confirmed seminal vesicle invasion, 14 were detected by the 3D TRUS, with a sensitivity, specificity, and PPV of 88%, 98%, and 98%, respectively.

An interesting study conducted by Sedelaar and colleagues [51] compared 3D gray-scale TRUS findings in 50 patients diagnosed with prostate cancer with findings in 50 patients diagnosed with BPH. The patients were analyzed by two blinded, independent radiologists. The 3D TRUS demonstrated a significantly greater sensitivity (88% versus 72%) than 2D TRUS, but decreased specificity (42% versus 54%) in identifying lesions suspicious for cancer in the two groups. However, since the improvement in cancer detection and staging is exclusively dependent on visualization of the lesion, isoechoic lesions were almost unanimously missed. The authors concluded that despite the increased sensitivity, 3D TRUS did not add to the detection and staging of prostate cancer, as compared with 2D TRUS.

Contrast-enhanced ultrasound of the prostate

Contrast-enhanced power Doppler angiography is another ultrasound-based technology for imaging of the prostate that is employed after intravenous administration of microbubbles. The microbubbles circulate throughout the body in the blood stream and enhance color Doppler contrast.

The majority of ultrasound contrast agents consist of gas-encapsulated microbubbles, with a diameter less than 10 μm. This allows the penetration of the microbubbles into the microvascular system. The half-life of these microbubbles is no longer than several minutes. At low energies the bubbles oscillate linearly, resulting in symmetrical compression and expansion phases. At intermediate energy levels the expansion and compression phases are not symmetrical. This allows the separation of reflected signals of tissue from the bubbles. At higher intensities the microbubbles will be disrupted. A high-intensity signal can be recorded and will result in enhanced Doppler imaging [52–55]. Twenty seconds after IV injection, an enhancement of the vascular system of the prostate can be detected. Halpern and colleagues [56] demonstrated significantly improved

sensitivity for detecting prostate cancer from 38% to 65%, with preserved specificity at approximately 80%. In another study of 18 patients undergoing prostate biopsies, Bogers and coworkers [57] found a significant increase in sensitivity from 35% to 85% with preserved specificity. Frauscher and colleagues [58] reported in a prospective study of 230 male volunteers that targeted biopsies based on contrast-enhanced color Doppler detected a number of tumors equal to that of systematic biopsies, with less than half the number of biopsies.

Goossen and coworkers [59] demonstrated that time to peak enhancement in the prostate was the most predictive parameter for the localization of a malignancy-containing area in the prostate. This allowed for a 78% correct diagnosis.

In a recent study by Halpren and colleagues [60], the authors reported on the detection and differentiation between BPH and prostate cancer with contrast-enhanced ultrasonography in 301 men referred for prostate biopsy. They underwent contrast-enhanced sonography using continuous harmonic imaging (CHI) and intermittent harmonic imaging (IHI), in addition to continuous color and power Doppler. Harmonic imaging involves detecting the secondary (or harmonic) frequencies reflected from objects struck by diagnostic ultrasound of the primary frequency emitted by the ultrasound probe. Targeted biopsy cores were obtained initially from sites with greatest enhancement. Thereafter, systematic sextant core biopsies were obtained. Malignancy was detected in 363 biopsies from 104 of 301 subjects (35%). Cancer was diagnosed in 15.5% (175 of 1133) of targeted cores and 10.4% (188 of 1806) of sextant cores ($P < .01$). In the subset of patients diagnosed with prostate cancer, targeted cores were twice as likely to be positive (odds ratio [OR] = 2.0, $P < .001$). Additionally, a statistically significant advantage was found for IHI over baseline imaging ($P < .05$). The authors concluded that the detection rate of malignancy in contrast-enhanced targeted cores is significantly higher than in sextant cores. Despite these promising results, contrast-enhanced Doppler ultrasound has not yet gained popularity because of its high costs and low specificity rate [61].

Therapeutic applications of ultrasound of the prostate

Focused ultrasound can be used in a variety of therapeutic applications. It has been established for many years that high-intensity focused ultrasound (HIFU) delivers high energy, causing rapid coagulation necrosis of tissue within the target area with minimal damage to the surrounding tissue. The first clinical attempts to use ultrasound for treatment were made almost half a century ago with the ablation of brain tissue. However, only in recent years, with the development of high-powered ultrasound arrays and noninvasive monitoring methods, have clinical applications become more widespread.

In the past decade, HIFU has been adapted and used to treat small renal tumors, testicular tumors, and localized prostate cancer [62]. However, the largest currently available clinical experience with HIFU therapy is for BPH and prostate cancer using transrectal HIFU devices. HIFU currently is available commercially for these indications, mainly in Europe. Early short-term results demonstrated that prostate HIFU is effective in achieving local control for low- and intermediate-risk localized prostate cancer [63].

Blana and colleagues [64] recently reported their 5-year results with transrectal HIFU in the treatment of localized prostate cancer in 146 patients with Stage T1–T2N0M0 prostate cancer. Prostate-specific antigen (PSA) levels of 15 ng/mL or less and a Gleason score of 7 or less were considered the inclusion criteria. Mean follow-up was 22.5 months (range 4 to 62 months) and included PSA measurement and control sextant biopsies. The median PSA nadir 3 months after HIFU treatment was 0.07 ng/mL (range 0 to 5.67 ng/mL). At a mean follow-up of 22 months, the median PSA level was 0.15 ng/mL (range 0 to 12.11 ng/mL); 87% of patients had a constant PSA level of less than 1 ng/mL; 93.4% of patients had negative follow-up biopsies. Although 12% of patients underwent TURP after HIFU due to obstruction, no severe stress incontinence (grade 2 to 3) was documented. Erectile function was preserved in 47.3% of patients, and the International Prostate Symptom Score and quality of life index before and after treatment were comparable. The authors concluded that HIFU is efficacious and has low levels of associated morbidity. It does not exclude other treatment options and is repeatable when necessary.

Long-term follow-up is required to validate the efficacy of prostate HIFU in terms of disease-free survival and overall mortality. Nonetheless, many consider HIFU a viable alternative treatment for patients that are poor candidates for radical prostatectomy.

References

[1] Engelbrecht MR, et al. Prostate cancer staging using imaging. BJU Int 2000;86(Suppl 1):123–34.

[2] Borley N, et al. Laparoscopic pelvic lymph node dissection allows significantly more accurate staging in "high-risk" prostate cancer compared to MRI or CT. Scand J Urol Nephrol 2003;37(5): 382–6.

[3] D'Amico AV, et al. Critical analysis of the ability of the endorectal coil magnetic resonance imaging scan to predict pathologic stage, margin status, and post-operative prostate-specific antigen failure in patients with clinically organ-confined prostate cancer. J Clin Oncol 1996;14(6):1770–7.

[4] Engelbrecht MR, et al. Local staging of prostate cancer using magnetic resonance imaging: a meta-analysis. Eur Radiol 2002;12(9):2294–302.

[5] Hendrikx AJ, et al. Ultrasonic determination of prostatic volume: a cadaver study. Urology 1989; 34(3):123–5.

[6] Aarnink RG, et al. Formula-derived prostate volume determination. Eur Urol 1996;29(4):399–402.

[7] Aarnink RG, et al. Planimetric volumetry of the prostate: how accurate is it? Physiol Meas 1995; 16(3):141–50.

[8] Salo JO, et al. Computerized tomography and trans-rectal ultrasound in the assessment of local extension of prostatic cancer before radical retropubic prostatectomy. J Urol 1987;137(3):435–8.

[9] Bates TS, et al. A comparison of endorectal magnetic resonance imaging and transrectal ultrasonography in the local staging of prostate cancer with histopathological correlation. Br J Urol 1997;79(6): 927–32.

[10] Presti JC Jr, et al. Local staging of prostatic carcinoma: comparison of transrectal sonography and endorectal MR imaging. AJR Am J Roentgenol 1996;166(1):103–8.

[11] Rifkin MD, et al. Comparison of magnetic resonance imaging and ultrasonography in staging early prostate cancer. Results of a multi-institutional cooperative trial. N Engl J Med 1990;323(10):621–6.

[12] Hardeman SW, et al. Transrectal ultrasound for staging prior to radical prostatectomy. Urology 1989;34(4):175–80.

[13] Augustin H, et al. Differences in biopsy features between prostate cancers located in the transition and peripheral zone. BJU Int 2003;91(6):477–81.

[14] Shinohara K, Wheeler TM, Scardino PT. The appearance of prostate cancer on transrectal ultrasonography: correlation of imaging and pathological examinations. J Urol 1989;142(1):76–82.

[15] Terris MK, McNeal JE, Stamey TA. Estimation of prostate cancer volume by transrectal ultrasound imaging. J Urol 1992;147(3 Pt 2):855–7.

[16] Okihara K, et al. Kinetic analysis of focal hypoechoic lesion in the prostate treated by castration. Prostate 1994;24(5):252–6.

[17] Watanabe H, Kojima M. The role of prostatic planimetry using transrectal sonography in prostatic diseases. Semin Surg Oncol 1997;13(6):425–30.

[18] Rifkin MD, Sudakoff GS, Alexander AA. Prostate: techniques, results, and potential applications of color Doppler US scanning. Radiology 1993; 186(2):509–13.

[19] Neumaier CE, et al. Normal prostate gland: examination with color Doppler US. Radiology 1995; 196(2):453–7.

[20] Kelly IM, Lees WR, Rickards D. Prostate cancer and the role of color Doppler US. Radiology 1993; 189(1):153–6.

[21] Patel U, Rickards D. The diagnostic value of colour Doppler flow in the peripheral zone of the prostate, with histological correlation. Br J Urol 1994;74(5): 590–5.

[22] Newman JS, Bree RL, Rubin JM. Prostate cancer: diagnosis with color Doppler sonography with histologic correlation of each biopsy site. Radiology 1995;195(1):86–90.

23 Bree RL. The role of color Doppler and staging biopsies in prostate cancer detection. Urology 1997;49(3A Suppl):31–4.

[24] Cornud F, et al. Color Doppler-guided prostate biopsies in 591 patients with an elevated serum PSA level: impact on Gleason score for nonpalpable lesions. Urology 1997;49(5):709–15.

[25] Lavoipierre AM, et al. Prostatic cancer: role of color Doppler imaging in transrectal sonography. AJR Am J Roentgenol 1998;171(1):205–10.

[26] Halpern EJ, et al. Prostate: high-frequency Doppler US imaging for cancer detection. Radiology 2002; 225(1):71–7.

[27] Rubin JM, et al. Power Doppler US: a potentially useful alternative to mean frequency-based color Doppler US. Radiology 1994;190(3):853–6.

[28] Murphy KJ, Rubin JM. Power Doppler: it's a good thing. Semin Ultrasound CT MR 1997;18(1):13–21.

[29] Tsuru N, et al. Role of Doppler ultrasound and resistive index in benign prostatic hypertrophy. Int J Urol 2002;9(8):427–30.

[30] Kojima M, et al. Preliminary results of power Doppler imaging in benign prostatic hyperplasia. Ultrasound Med Biol 1997;23(9):1305–9.

[31] Kojima M, et al. Doppler resistive index in benign prostatic hyperplasia: correlation with ultrasonic appearance of the prostate and infravesical obstruction. Eur Urol 2000;37(4):436–42.

[32] Leventis AK, et al. Characteristics of normal prostate vascular anatomy as displayed by power Doppler. Prostate 2001;46(4):281–8.

[33] Tsuru N, et al. Resistance index in benign prostatic hyperplasia using power Doppler imaging and clinical outcomes after transurethral vaporization of the prostate. Int J Urol 2005;12(3):264–9.

[34] Siegal J, Brawer MK. Significance of neovascularity in human prostate carcinoma. In: Foster C, Bostwick DG, editors. Pathology of the prostate:

major problems in pathology, Vol. 34. Philadelphia: Saunders; 1998. p. xvii, 443, [4] of plates.

[35] Brawer MK, et al. Predictors of pathologic stage in prostatic carcinoma. The role of neovascularity. Cancer 1994;73(3):678–87.

[36] Gasparini G, Harris A. Prognostic significance of tumor vascularity. In: Teicher BA, editor. Antiangiogenic agents in cancer therapy. Totowa, NJ: Humana Press; 1999. p. xi, 450.

[37] Evans SM, et al. Use of power Doppler ultrasound-guided biopsies to locate regions of tumour hypoxia. Br J Cancer 1997;76(10):1308–14.

[38] Potdevin TC, et al. Doppler quantitative measures by region to discriminate prostate cancer. Ultrasound Med Biol 2001;27(10):1305–10.

[39] Hall MC, et al. Significance of tumor angiogenesis in clinically localized prostate carcinoma treated with external beam radiotherapy. Urology 1994;44(6):869–75.

[40] Gee MS, et al. Doppler ultrasound imaging detects changes in tumor perfusion during antivascular therapy associated with vascular anatomic alterations. Cancer Res 2001;61(7):2974–82.

[41] Cornud F, et al. Endorectal color doppler sonography and endorectal MR imaging features of nonpalpable prostate cancer: correlation with radical prostatectomy findings. AJR Am J Roentgenol 2000;175(4):1161–8.

[42] Halpern EJ, et al. High-frequency Doppler US of the prostate: effect of patient position. Radiology 2002; 222(3):634–9.

[43] Okihara K, Miki T, Joseph Babaian R. Clinical efficacy of prostate cancer detection using power doppler imaging in American and Japanese men. J Clin Ultrasound 2002;30(4):213–21.

[44] Arger PH, et al. Color and power Doppler sonography in the diagnosis of prostate cancer: comparison between vascular density and total vascularity. J Ultrasound Med 2004;23(5):623–30.

[45] Hsing AW, Tsao L, Devesa SS. International trends and patterns of prostate cancer incidence and mortality. Int J Cancer 2000;85(1):60–7.

[46] Ellis WJ, et al. Diagnosis of prostatic carcinoma: the yield of serum prostate specific antigen, digital rectal examination and transrectal ultrasonography. J Urol 1994;152(5 Pt 1):1520–5.

[47] Carter HB, et al. Evaluation of transrectal ultrasound in the early detection of prostate cancer. J Urol 1989;142(4):1008–10.

[48] Hamper UM, et al. Three-dimensional US of the prostate: early experience. Radiology 1999;212(3): 719–23.

[49] Garg S, et al. Staging of prostate cancer using 3-dimensional transrectal ultrasound images: a pilot study. J Urol 1999;162(4):1318–21.

[50] Strasser H, et al. Three-dimensional transrectal ultrasound in staging of localised prostate cancer. J Urol 2003;169(Supp 4):299 [A.].

[51] Sedelaar JP, et al. Three-dimensional grayscale ultrasound: evaluation of prostate cancer compared

with benign prostatic hyperplasia. Urology 2001; 57(5):914–20.

[52] Chomas JE, et al. Mechanisms of contrast agent destruction. IEEE Trans Ultrason Ferroelectr Freq Control 2001;48(1):232–48.

[53] Dayton P, et al. Optical and acoustical observations of the effects of ultrasound on contrast agents. IEEE Trans Ultrason Ferroelectr Freq Control 1999;46:220–32.

[54] Kamiyama N, et al. Analysis of flash echo from contrast agent for designing optimal ultrasound diagnostic systems. Ultrasound Med Biol 1999;25(3):411–20.

[55] Tiemann K, et al. Stimulated acoustic emission: pseudo-Doppler shifts seen during the destruction of nonmoving microbubbles. Ultrasound Med Biol 2000;26(7):1161–7.

[56] Halpern EJ, Rosenberg M, Gomella LG. Prostate cancer: contrast-enhanced US for detection. Radiology 2001;219(1):219–25.

[57] Bogers HA, Sedelaar JPM, Beerlage HP, et al. Contrast-enhanced three-dimensional power Doppler angiography of the human prostate: correlation with biopsy outcome. Urology 1999;54:97–104.

[58] Frauscher F, et al. Comparison of contrast enhanced color Doppler targeted biopsy with conventional systematic biopsy: impact on prostate cancer detection. J Urol 2002;167(4):1648–52.

[59] Goossen T, et al. The value of dynamic contrast enhanced power Doppler ultrasound in the localization of prostate carcinoma. Eur Urol 2002;1(Supp 1):91.

[60] Halpern EJ, et al. Detection of prostate carcinoma with contrast-enhanced sonography using intermittent harmonic imaging. Cancer 2005;104(11):2373–83.

[61] Pepe P, et al. Does the adjunct of ecographic contrast medium Levovist improve the detection rate of prostate cancer? Prostate Cancer Prostatic Dis 2003;6(2):159–62.

[62] Madersbacher S, Marberger M. High-energy shockwaves and extracorporeal high-intensity focused ultrasound. J Endourol 2003;17(8):667–72.

[63] Colombel M, Gelet A. Principles and results of high-intensity focused ultrasound for localized prostate cancer. Prostate Cancer Prostatic Dis 2004;7(4):289–94.

[64] Blana A, et al. High-intensity focused ultrasound for the treatment of localized prostate cancer: 5-year experience. Urology 2004;63(2):297–300.

ELSEVIER
SAUNDERS

Urol Clin N Am 33 (2006) 339–352

UROLOGIC
CLINICS
of North America

Imaging Associated with Percutaneous and Intraoperative Management of Renal Tumors

J. Kyle Anderson, MD[a,b], W. Bruce Shingleton, MD[c],
Jeffrey A. Cadeddu, MD[d,*]

[a]Department of Urology, The University of Minnesota, Mayo Memorial Building, 420 Delaware Street Southeast,
Room A597, Minneapolis, MN 55455, USA
[b]The Veterans Affairs Medical Center, 1 Veterans Drive, Minneapolis, MN 55417, USA
[c]Department of Urology, The Louisiana State University Health Sciences Center, 1501 Kings Highway,
Shreveport, LA 71103, USA
[d]Department of Urology, The University of Texas Southwestern Medical Center, 5323 Harry Hines Boulevard,
Dallas, TX 75390, USA

Technologic advances are changing the way renal tumors are diagnosed and treated. Widespread use of CT for evaluating abdominal symptoms has allowed renal tumors to be diagnosed while at a small size, with many tumors now discovered incidentally before the onset of symptoms or metastatic disease [1]. The increased prevalence of smaller tumors led initially to the development and preference for open partial nephrectomy to preserve renal function. At the same time, advances in laparoscopy offered an entirely new treatment option with a marked reduction in postoperative morbidity and more rapid convalescence. Currently, laparoscopic partial nephrectomy (LPN) is the preferred, yet technically demanding, nephron-sparing option.

To further reduce the morbidity of these procedures, ablative treatment for renal tumors has been developed. Cryoablation (CA) and radiofrequency ablation (RFA) are the two primary modalities in clinical use. Both procedures can be performed laparoscopically or percutaneously, and together these treatments offer numerous advantages over other alternatives. Not only are these procedures less technically demanding that LPN, but the morbidity, especially following the

percutaneous modalities, is further reduced even relative to LPN.

Although these advantages have been an improvement in patient care, thermally based ablative technologies have presented new challenges to the practicing urologist. With traditional extirpative renal procedures (radical or partial nephrectomy), excision is under direct visual guidance by the surgeon, and the margin of excision is confirmed by pathological examination of the specimen. During an ablative, especially percutaneous, procedure, the role of direct visual guidance is reduced greatly and reliance instead is placed on image guidance technologies, including ultrasonography, CT, or MRI. Additionally, by leaving the ablated tissue in place, pathologic verification of complete tumor ablation is not possible. Although biopsy has been used in an attempt to confirm ablation, this technique has not proven reliable given the inherent false-negative rate associated with random needle sampling.

Given this situation, cross-sectional imaging must be used to answer a new question: has an ablation been successful and caused total cell death within the desired treatment zone? Although current follow-up recommendations for a T1 renal cell carcinoma resected by means of partial nephrectomy include only yearly chest radiograph and physical examination with no imaging of the kidneys [2], the new ablative treatments present a distinctly different situation.

---

* Corresponding author.
E-mail address: jeffrey.cadeddu@utsouthwestern.edu (J.A. Cadeddu).

Given that long-term follow-up is not yet available, and pathologic verification of resection is not possible, follow-up assessment of the ablated tumor needs to be performed. Obviously, following ablative treatment, the determination of cellular viability within a defined anatomic area is a new imaging challenge compared with the more traditional roles of anatomical differentiation or procedural guidance. Unfortunately, the ideal imaging modality to simultaneously provide anatomic information and cellular viability data does not exist. Because the success of these new ablation technologies relies not only on the technology itself but also the advantages and limitations of the associated radiographic techniques to achieve success, it is critical for urologic surgeons employing CA or RFA to understand how to use and interpret radiographic imaging. Thus this article describes both the intraoperative imaging needed for ablation targeting and guidance and the postablation radiographic follow-up that is critical to achieving a successful outcome.

Intraoperative imaging—laparoscopic partial nephrectomy

Before discussing the imaging requirements and issues associated with CA or RFA, it should be emphasized that imaging also plays a critical role in the intraoperative approach to laparoscopic partial nephrectomy. Given the limited exposure and tactile sensation offered by a laparoscopic approach, ultrasonography is used to better delineate normal parenchyma from renal tumor. Typically this is done using a laparoscopic ultrasound probe after removal of Gerota's fascia and the peri-renal fat surrounding, but not overlying, the tumor. Examination of the tumor from multiple angles provides the surgeon with a thorough understanding of tumor depth, size, and relationship to the collecting system and renal vasculature. Presence of satellite lesions may be identified also [3]. Recently, Nguyen and colleagues developed a technique using ultrasound-guided needle localization of deep tumor margin to further differentiate the extent of a renal tumor [4]. In experienced hands, however, ultrasound guidance alone for LPN has been helpful in maintaining low margin rates (3% to 3.5%) and successful oncologic outcomes [5,6]. The main challenge for the operating surgeon is familiarity with ultrasonographic anatomy and image interpretation and manipulation of the laparoscopic

ultrasound probe. With the assistance of a radiologist and practice, however, informative surgical images are attainable.

Intraoperative imaging—cryoablation

Laparoscopic renal cryoablation requires the use of a flexible laparoscopic ultrasound transducer. The use of this devise is very important for the accurate placement of the cryoprobes in the tumor and iceball monitoring. Laparoscopic ultrasound requires surgeon familiarity with device manipulation and image interpretation. Early in the surgeon's experience, intraoperative participation of a radiologist is recommended. The cryoprobes (17 gauge IceRod, Oncura, Plymouth Meeting, PA) usually are placed in a triangular configuration under ultrasound guidance for tumors less than 3.5 cm in diameter. The ideal spacing interval is 1.5 cm between probe locations. Larger tumors may require more probes, but again the spacing requirement is 1.5 cm apart. During the initial freezing cycle, the progress of the iceball is monitored by ultrasound. The ice front is extended to 10 mm beyond the tumor border. It is critical that the ultrasound probe is positioned such that a clear image of the deep parenchymal margin of the tumor is visualized. This often requires mobilization of all or most of the kidney. The surgeon must be able to image the iceball from multiple perspectives to ensure complete tumor coverage, because only the ice front closest to the probe is visualized (Fig. 1). If the entire iceball is not visualized, the surgeon risks incomplete ablation. An active thaw cycle then is undertaken with ultrasound monitoring of the thaw. After this is complete, a second freeze cycle is initiated. If there are any critical structures such as the renal artery or vein, care should be taken to monitor the icefront with ultrasound. Upon completion of the second freeze cycle, a passive thaw, which does not require ultrasound monitoring, is performed.

Intraoperative imaging—radiofrequency ablation

Laparoscopic approach

During laparoscopic RFA, the primary mode of guidance is visual. For exophytic tumors, a multi-tine electrode (eg, Starburst XL, RITA Medical Systems, Fremont, CA) is preferred, because the individual tines can be deployed fully and visually confirmed to protrude through the

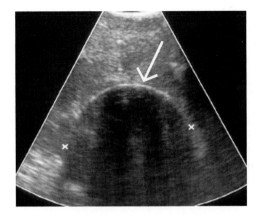

Fig. 1. Transverse laparoscopic ultrasound on renal surface opposite kidney tumor shows curvilinear hypere-
chogenic interface with posterior shadowing. Arrow
denotes iceball margin enveloping entire tumor (not
seen because of shadowing). (*Reproduced from* Remer
EM, Hale JC, O'Malley CM, et al. Sonographic guidance of laparoscopic renal cryoablation. AJR Am J
Roent 2000;174(6):1595–6; with permission.)

capsule of a tumor. The tines then can be drawn in
(shrink ablation zone) to the tumor edge under direct visual guidance. In this position, the surgeon
can confidently ablate the tumor with a 5 mm
margin. For more endophytic tumors, ultrasonography is helpful, as it provides information on tumor size and depth similar to LPN. In these cases,
the tines of a multi-tined electrode are visualized
on ultrasonography as they traverse the tumor,
and tine location can be confirmed 0.5 to 1.0 cm
beyond the renal tumor periphery. If a single
probe design is employed, ultrasonography is
used to identify the probe as it traverses the tumor
to the deep margin.

Ultrasonography is not effective in confirming
the extent of ablation. In both animal models [7]
and human renal tumors [8], RFA creates an
area of heterogeneous echotexture with some hy-
perechogenicity, yet this area does not correlate
to the size of the final lesion. Improved correlation
between ultrasonography results and final ablation size has been achieved in a porcine model using contrast-enhanced three-dimensional
ultrasound [9,10]. Johnson and colleagues were
able to correlate contrast-enhanced ultrasound
measurements of RFA lesions to within 0.3 cm
of the final pathologic lesion size in 16 swine,
but this technique has yet to be well-studied in
people. Real-time imaging of the ablation, however, is not necessary, because the deployed tine
diameter defines the final ablation diameter.

Percutaneous radiofrequency ablation

Ultrasound, MRI, and CT have been used for
guidance of percutaneously placed RF electrodes.
Given the limited resolution of ultrasonography
and the limited availability of procedure-capable
MRIs, CT has been the most frequently used
modality for this technique, although MRI guidance is feasible [11]. The three-dimensional view
provided by CT can identify a percutaneous route
to the tumor that will avoid surrounding structures such as bowel, spleen, liver, or pleura. Further, imaging can be used to confirm individual
tine placement (for a multi-tine electrode) to ensure ablation 0.5 to 1.0 cm beyond the renal tumor periphery. Immediate postablation contrast-
enhanced imaging also is able to confirm lack of
enhancement within the ablation zone consistent
with a successful ablation. Ultrasonography guidance is not recommended, as it clearly provides inferior tissue resolution, tine/probe placement, and
three-dimensional imaging. In addition, ultrasonography cannot be used to assess immediate
post-treatment success.

Imaging following cryoablation

There are two mechanisms that cause tumor
destruction during the freeze process: direct cell
injury and vascular injury. These occur as the result
of the temperature in the tumor reaching −20°
to −40°C, which is the lethal temperature required
for cell destruction. An important point to understand is that the leading edge of the ice front is
0°C, which will result in only sublethal cellular
injury. It is therefore necessary to extend the ice
front 5 to 10 mm beyond the tumor border to
ensure that total cellular destruction occurs. The
sublethal injury zone appears as a hypervascular
ring surrounding the cryolesion in some patients
on postcryoimaging studies [12]. This finding will
be discussed in greater detail later.

What follow-up modality best assesses total
tumor destruction? Some investigators have used
percutaneous biopsy after cryosurgery for assessing tumor destruction. Chen and colleagues
reported on 35 patients who underwent laparoscopic renal CA [13]. Twenty-one of the patients
underwent CT-guided biopsies at 3 or 6 months
after CA. All biopsies were negative for residual
tumor and only demonstrated fibrosis and hemo-
siderin deposits. Nadler and colleagues reported
on 15 patients who had laparoscopic renal CA
performed [14]. Seven of 10 patients who had

renal cell carcinoma underwent percutaneous biopsy 3 months after procedure, with two of the seven biopsies positive for residual tumor. Cestari and colleagues described their results in 35 patients who underwent laparoscopic renal cryosurgery [15]. CT-guided biopsies were performed in 25 patients at 6 month follow-up, with all biopsies negative for neoplasm. From these studies, it appears that most patients undergoing renal CA have no evidence of residual tumor on repeat biopsy.

As noted earlier, however, studies have shown limited accuracy for renal tumor biopsy. One difficulty in reliance on post-CA biopsies for determination of tumor ablation is the reported 19% false-negative rate for needle biopsies performed directly into surgically exposed renal tumors [16]. Needle aspiration is even less successful, as Campbell and colleagues found a 25% false-negative rate in 25 patients who underwent needle aspiration of a renal mass [17]. Additionally, Cestari and colleagues reported one patient who had a negative post-CA biopsy but subsequently had a suspicious lesion on follow-up MRI and was found to have renal carcinoma [15]. Thus, if a biopsy is obtained and demonstrates no viable tumor present, radiographic follow-up remains necessary.

There are four imaging modalities available to evaluate tumor responses to CA. These include ultrasonography CT, MRI, and positron emission tomography (PET) scans. PET technology is not sufficiently developed to allow accurate assessment of tumor destruction after CA or RFA, and it is not recommended for routine surveillance imaging. Ultrasonography is useful in documenting changes in linear size but is limited in its ability to assess the presence of viable tumor. There has been a recent report on the use of contrast-enhanced harmonic ultrasound for

tumor evaluation after CA. Zhu and colleagues described the ultrasound findings in three patients who underwent renal CA [18]. Using contrast-enhanced ultrasound, decreased enhancement was seen similar to that present on post-CA CT scans. One case of persistent enhancement was identified that was related to a local recurrence. Further evaluation in a larger series of patients would be required to determine the feasibility and reproducibility of this technique. Thus CT and MRI are the preferred modalities for post-CA surveillance.

There has been no commonly accepted time interval to obtain postablation imaging studies. In early studies investigating CA, MR scans were obtained on postablation day 1 [19]. Typically, these scans only showed hemorrhage with perfusion defects and were limited by postprocedure hemorrhage. There is no reason to obtain a post-CA scan until a minimum of 1 month has lapsed to allow for resolution of any possible hemorrhage (WB Shingleton, unpublished data). Some investigators obtain the first scan at 3 to 6 months, and if this scan demonstrates no enhancement, biannual scans are obtained [13,14,19]. The authors' recommendation is to obtain an imaging study at 1, 3, and 6 months. If the lesion is nonenhancing and stable in size, biannual studies are obtained. In cases where the lesion has regressed completely, annual scans are satisfactory.

Characteristics of ablation zone

CT imaging provides the opportunity to assess for the presence of viable tumor post-CA. In order for this to be achieved, an unenhanced scan of the kidneys with thin 3 mm slices must be performed first. Intravenous contrast then is administered and subsequent scanning undertaken. The typical radiographic appearance of the cryolesion is that of nonenhancement. Fig. 2 illustrates a renal

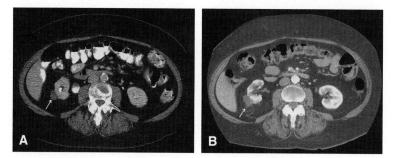

Fig. 2. (*A*) Exophytic enhancing right posterior lateral renal mass—precryoablation (*arrow*). (*B*) Nonenhancement of renal mass immediately after cryoablation (*arrow*).

tumor before and after CA on contrast-enhanced scans. It is an absolute requirement that no enhancement occur in the cryolesion for the treatment to be considered successful. Any evidence of enhancement indicates there is residual tumor present that will require further treatment. In some circumstances, the cryolesion may have a larger diameter than the original tumor because of some hemorrhage secondary to probe insertion. Alternatively, the iceball may have been extended beyond the tumor border. This should not be a concern, but rather expected, as long as there is no enhancement present. Evidence of nonenhancement (less than 10 to 12 Hounsfield units on CT) in the ablated tumor is the key definition of complete tumor destruction. Rodriquez and colleagues reported their results of laparoscopic renal cryosurgery in seven patients in whom contrast-enhanced CT scans were performed at 3 to 6 month intervals and demonstrated perfusion defects at the ablated area with some tumor shrinkage [20]. Lee and colleagues described their results in 20 patients after laparoscopic renal cryotherapy and at a mean follow-up of 14.2 months; no ablated masses demonstrated residual enhancement in CT or MRI scans [21]. It has been documented that patients with residual enhancement in the cryolesion who subsequently undergo biopsy will be found to have residual disease (WB Shingleton, unpublished data) [23].

Another factor to be evaluated on post-treatment CT images is the size of the lesion. The tumor should demonstrate a decrease in size as seen on cross-sectional imaging as early as 3 months after treatment [22]. This most likely occurs as the result of a cellular response to CA in which an acute neutrophil reaction stimulates macrophage activity and absorption of lysed

cellular debris [23]. This leads to a decrease in size of the tumor along with fibrosis formation. Gill and colleagues in their initial series of patients reported that 20% of their patients had complete disappearance of the lesion [19]. Eleven of 15 tumors in Nadler's series decreased in size during the 6- to 72-month follow-up period [14]. Thus, shrinkage in tumor size appears to occur over a 6- to 12-month time period after ablation. The key point is that if there is any increase in size during follow-up, the possibility of a tumor recurrence should be considered, and a biopsy of the lesion recommended. The authors have treated one patient who had a lesion that was nonenhancing but increasing in size and who was found to have tumor recurrence after CA.

Fig. 3 illustrates the typical shrinkage of a tumor after CA with only a small amount of nonenhancing scar seen at 1 year follow-up. In some cases, the tumor will be reabsorbed completely, and there will be no visualization seen on follow-up imaging. The case in Fig. 4 additionally illustrates a common occurrence seen post-CA, which is the presence of a small periablation hemorrhage. These hemorrhages are seen typically in scans obtained early after the ablation procedure (1 day to 1 month). The hemorrhage can obscure clear visualization of the cryolesion, requiring repetition of the scan in 1 to 2 months to allow accurate assessment.

MRI has been used for post-CA imaging by some investigators [13,14]. The use of MRI is mandated in some clinical settings, such as in patients with compromised renal function or contrast allergy for whom the use of contrast would be contraindicated. If a patient has decreased kidney function, obtaining an unenhanced CT scan is unsatisfactory for the evaluation of tumor

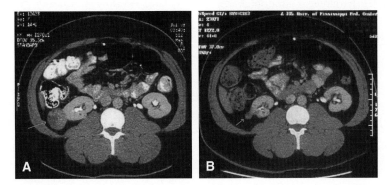

Fig. 3. (A) Right posterior lateral renal tumor precryoablation (arrows). (B) Fibrotic remnant of tumor postablation at 1 year—no enhancement (arrows).

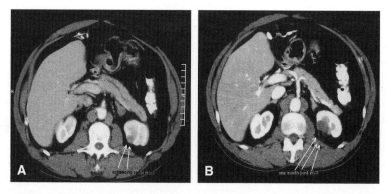

Fig. 4. (*A*) Precryoablation CT scan with left medial parenchymal tumor (*arrows*). (*B*) Intraparenchymal hemorrhage at 1 month obscuring ablated tumor (*arrows*).

ablation. Remer and colleagues first described the MR imaging characteristics of a cryolesion over time in 21 patients [12]. T1, T2, and T1 gadolinium-enhanced images were obtained at day 1 after CA, then 1, 3, 6, and 12 months after the procedure. In the 1- and 3-month scans, most of T1 images were isotense, and T2 images were mainly hypointense and without enhancement. Approximately 30% of lesions had a thin or thick rim of enhancement noted on the T1-enhanced images (Fig. 5). The 6- and 12-month scans showed T1 images to be isotense, and T2 images mainly hypo- or isotense, with no enhancement in T1 gadolinium images. The peripheral rim enhancement, which had been noted at 3 and 6 months, had resolved by 12 months. Fig. 6 illustrates a small inferior pole lesion before and after CA on MR images. As noted on the T1 enhanced postablation image, the lesion had regressed in

size almost completely. Remer noted that in 12 patients with 12-month follow-up, the cryolesion size decreased from 74% to 100% [12]. Additionally, perinephric changes were visualized in the scans at 1 and 3 months, with increased signal intensity in T2 images consistent with fluid accumulation. Nadler and colleagues reported that 13 of 15 their patients were imaged with MR post-CA [14]. All lesions were noted to be stable or decreasing in size with no enhancement.

Local recurrences following cryoablation

The appearance of residual or recurrent tumor on CT imaging is characterized by enhancement on postcontrast scans. Residual tumor can be noted typically on the first post-CA scan obtained at 1 or 3 months (Fig. 7). Local recurrences have been reported to occur up to 3 years after ablation; therefore, long-term follow-up is required. Typically, a recurrence is characterized by a new enhancing portion of the original ablated tumor adjacent to or surrounded by the nonenhancing ablated defect. Fig. 8 demonstrates a central recurrence 3 years after undergoing CA. Pathologic examination of this case demonstrated a 2.0 cm renal cell carcinoma surrounded by fibrotic scar tissue.

On MRI, residual tumor after CA demonstrates a hyperintense signal on the T1 gadolinium scan (Fig. 9). Any evidence of enhancement in the region of the cryolesion, excluding a peripheral rim, should be considered viable tumor. Experience has shown that MRI is a completely acceptable method of imaging the cryolesion. Difficulty, however, can occur when follow-up MRI scans are not preformed at the same facility using the same scanner. The software required for imaging

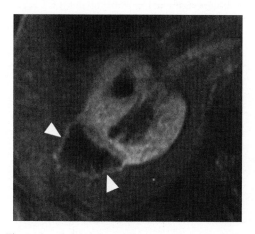

Fig. 5. A peripheral rim enhancement after cryoablation sometimes seen on postablation MR scans (*arrow heads*).

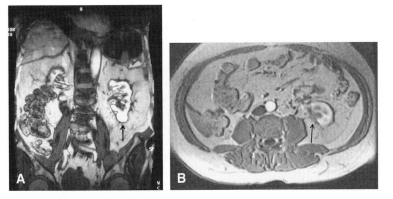

Fig. 6. (*A*) Precryoablation MR scan of exophytic left lower pole tumor (*arrow*)—T1 weighted image. (*B*) Four months postablation MR scan with almost complete regression of left medial lower pole tumor—T1 weighted image (*arrow*).

varies according to the different capabilities of each MRI unit. Therefore, there is no standard scanning technique used for MRI imaging of the kidney [24]. If MRI is used as the primary modality for monitoring of the post-CA lesion, it is important that the same unit and scanning technique be employed.

Imaging following radiofrequency ablation

Similar to CA, imaging options following RFA include ultrasonography, MRI, PET, and CT. Ultrasonography, while often the cheapest and most readily available modality, does not provide the sensitivity required for follow-up of ablated renal tumors. PET, while a promising modality, has not been well-investigated following RFA. MRI has adequate sensitivity for diagnosis of recurrent lesions, but the added cost inherent to MRI is a concern given the frequency of follow-up. MRI is necessary, however, for patients

unable to easily receive iodinated contrast agents because of renal failure or contrast allergy. In this regard, MRI, especially with gadolinium enhancement, is far superior to nonenhanced CT, whose use should be discouraged following RFA. Contrast-enhanced CT is the preferred imaging modality following RFA [25–30].

The optimal imaging interval following RFA has not been determined. Gervais and colleagues found day of the procedure CT images to underestimate final lesion size in one patient before abandoning this regimen [8]. At 1 week following ablation, Rendon and colleagues noted that only one of three patients with viable tumor had evidence of contrast enhancement [31]. Whether this lack of sensitivity at 1 week following ablation was a result of the study timing, inadequate sensitivity of CT, or difficulty of histologic analysis to determine viability of tissue [32], is unclear. Because of these findings, however, most authors

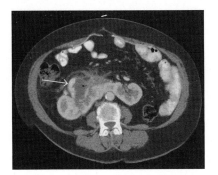

Fig. 7. Residual enhancing renal tumor after cryoablation (*arrow*).

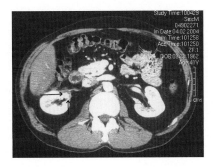

Fig. 8. Central recurrence of right medial tumor 3 years after cryoablation (*arrows*). Pathologic examination demonstrated a 2.0 cm renal cell carcinoma surrounded by fibrotic scar tissue.

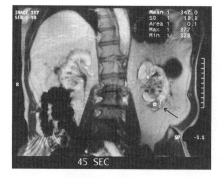

Fig. 9. Seven month postcryoablation T1 weighted post-gadolinium image demonstrating peripheral enhancement of left lower pole tumor (*arrow*).

have used a program with the first postprocedure imaging at 4 to 8 weeks after ablation, with subsequent tests performed at 3- to 6-month intervals. The authors' regimen is a follow-up study 6 weeks after ablation and then every 6 months. Using this surveillance schedule in their series of over 140 ablated renal tumors, the authors have encountered only one episode of metastasis. As evidence to the sensitivity of radiographic surveillance, however, this patient had been identified as having an incomplete ablation at his 6 week scan but was not retreated because of patient request. Regarding tapering of follow-up, renal CA and RFA are relatively new procedures, and it is not clear what the long-term protocol should be.

To fully understand radiologic follow-up after RFA, three characteristics of post-RFA imaging are important to highlight. First, incomplete ablations do occur, yet when identified, the patient can be retreated with little additional morbidity. Thus, the first scan following RFA must be scrutinized to identify evidence of untreated tumor. Second, as with CA, comparison of current to previous studies is a requirement, as recurrent lesions can be subtle and only identified because of their change with time. Thus, a thorough understanding of the normal radiological progression following RFA is required. Finally, as with CA, recurrences have occurred years after treatment, making continued surveillance prudent, and emphasizing the ability to recognize a recurrent tumor.

Initial assessment following radiofrequency ablation

Whether CT or MRI is used, the presence of contrast enhancement within the desired ablation zone suggests an incomplete ablation. On CT, contrast enhancement is defined as a greater than 10 to 12 Hounsfield units increase in enhancement following contrast administration. Theoretically, the periphery of the ablation zone is the most likely region for this to occur, especially on the edge abutting renal parenchyma as the heat sink provided by the highly vascularized parenchyma increases the likelihood of sublethal temperatures.

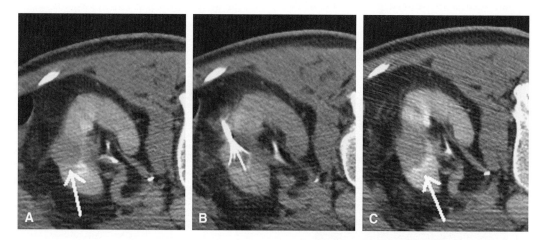

Fig. 10. Intraoperative radiofrequency ablation CT scans of a left-sided laterally located renal tumor. (*A*) Preablation image shows enhancing renal tumor (*arrow*). (*B*) Percutaneously placed multi-tine RF electrode is seen within the tumor. Additional images (not shown) confirm total coverage of lesion with tines extending beyond the tumor periphery. (*C*) Postablation image reveals lack of enhancement within the tumor suggesting a successful ablation (*arrow*).

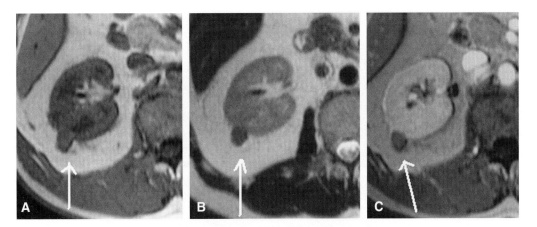

Fig. 11. Preoperative MRI before successful RFA of a right renal tumor. Tumor is isointense to renal parenchyma on T1-WI (*A—arrow*) and hypointense on T2-WI (*B—arrow*). It shows mild enhancement on postcontrast T1-WI (*C—arrow*). (*From* Svatek RS, Sims R, Anderson JK, et al. Magnetic resonance imaging characteristics of renal tumors following radiofrequency ablation. Urology 2006;67(3):508–12; with permission.)

With MRI, the detection of enhancement for CA and RFA can be more technique-dependent. Svatek and colleagues noted that occasionally tumor contrast enhancement of renal tumors on MRI may be almost visually imperceptible and only evident by intensity measurement [33]. They suggested this is caused by washout of contrast material before image acquisition and suggested multiple rapid acquisitions immediately following gadolinium administration to reveal early enhancement and the following washout. Regardless, the presence of enhancement within the desired ablation zone, whether on CT or MRI, at initial assessment following ablation suggests incomplete ablation and the need for additional treatment. Figs. 10 to 13 demonstrate the CT and MRI appearances before and following successful ablations of biopsy-proven renal tumors. Figs. 14 to 16 demonstrate incomplete ablations on initial treatment. Further treatment was required for these patients.

In addition to the lack of enhancement, a characteristic MRI pattern is seen following RFA. Svatek and colleagues examined post-RFA

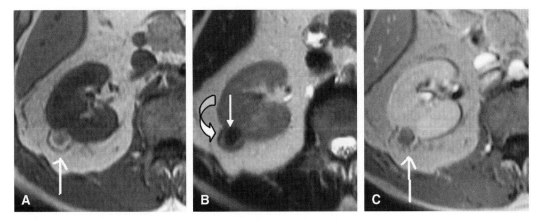

Fig. 12. MRI scans of tumor from Figure 11, 6 weeks following successful ablation. Ablation zone (*straight arrows*) is characterized by high signal intensity on T1-WI (*A*), very low SI on T2-WI (*B*), and lack of enhancement on postcontrast T1-WI (*C*). Peritumoral halo characteristic of percutaneously ablated lesions is seen as a rim of low signal intensity on T1 and T2 weighted images surrounding a zone of perinephric fat just external to the ablated area (*curved arrow*). (*From* Svatek RS, Sims R, Anderson JK, et al. Magnetic resonance imaging characteristics of renal tumors following radiofrequency ablation. Urology 2006;67(3):508–12; with permission.)

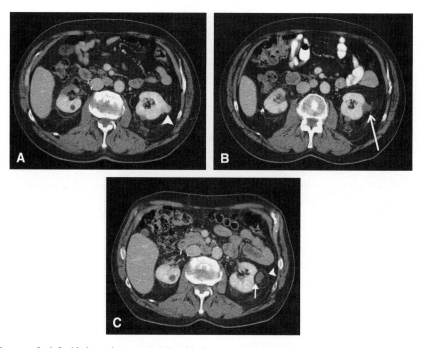

Fig. 13. CT scans of a left-sided renal tumor. (*A*) Preablation scan with white arrowhead highlighting enhancing tumor. (*B*) Scan 6 weeks after ablation. Note lack of enhancement at tumor (*arrow*). (*C*) Scan 30 months after ablation. Note the fat infiltration between the ablated tumor and kidney (*white arrow*) and the halo in the peri-tumor fat (*white arrow head*). (*From* Anderson JK, Matsumoto E, Cadeddu JA. Renal radio-frequency ablation: technique and results. Urol Oncol 2005;23(5):355–60; with permission.)

MRI images from 12 patients to better understand the lesion characteristics on this imaging modality [33]. On T1-weighted images (WI), all successfully treated tumors had high signal intensity (SI), but in 70%, there was significant heterogeneity in SI. Alternatively, on T2-WI, all successfully ablated tumors had low SI, and there was slight heterogeneity again in 70% of tumors. On MRI, these characteristics can provide additional information regarding extent of ablation.

The final radiologic finding encountered immediately after percutaneous but not laparoscopically guided RFA is the peri-tumor halo. A peri-tumor halo (seen as a rim of low SI on T1-WI and T2-WI) can be found in 71% of patients evaluated with MRI [33] and is frequently seen on CT following RFA (Figs. 12, 13) [34]. This halo likely represents scarring and fibrosis of the fatty tissue and fascia included in the ablation zone and should not be confused with tumor growth or angiomyolipoma. It is unique to percutaneous treatment, because Gerota's fat and fascia are cleared from the kidney before laparoscopic-guided ablation. This halo is frequently visible immediately following ablation, and it becomes more pronounced with time.

Changes in the ablated zone with time following radiofrequency ablation

As noted earlier, CA causes cell lysis followed by an acute neutrophil response, increased macrophage activity, and subsequent resorption of the tissue leading to a decrease in lesion size [23,35]. In contrast, acutely following RFA protein denaturation results in maintenance of cellular architecture [36]. Chronically, a granulomatous process with foreign body giant cell reaction predominates [37]. Because of this difference in post-ablation histopathology, significant reabsorption is not expected after RFA. Matsumoto and colleagues reviewed CT scans of 64 renal tumors taken over a median of 13.7 months after RFA (percutaneous and laparoscopic) and found an insignificant change in lesion size ($p = .68$) [34]. Gervais and colleagues had similar findings on CT follow-up with only 3 of 23 RFA-treated tumors decreasing in size [28]. On MRI, Svatek and colleagues encountered comparable results with mean lesion size decreasing from 2.65 to 2.4 cm at 12 months. Again, this change was not significant ($p = .54$) [33].

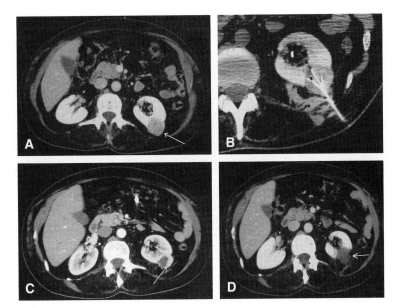

Fig. 14. CT scans of a left-sided posterior renal tumor. (*A*) Preablation scan revealing enhancing tumor (*arrow*). (*B*) Percutaneously placed multi-tine radiofrequency (RF) electrode is seen within the tumor. Additional images (not shown) suggest total coverage of lesion with electrode tines. (*C*) Scan 6 weeks after ablation reveals enhancement at periphery of tumor (*arrow*). (*D*) Scan at 6 weeks following reablation of the lesion. Note that after the second ablation there is no contrast enhancement within the renal tumor (*arrow*).

In addition to stability of ablation zone size, further evolutionary characteristics are expected from RFA lesions with time. Most importantly, any contrast enhancement appearing at a time distant from the ablation remains a sign of recurrence. This occurred in 1 of 64 (1.5%) tumors in Matsumoto's series and 0 of 12 tumors in the Svatek series [33,34]. Next, the peri-tumor halo seen on MRI and CT surrounding percutaneously treated RF lesions persists for most patients.

Regarding SI on MRI, Svatek and colleagues found that the initially high SI with significant heterogeneity on T1-WI and low SI with slight heterogeneity on T2-WI remain constant on long-term follow-up. Finally, on CT, there was a characteristic progression in lesion shape and relation to normal renal parenchyma with time. For endophytic tumors, the initial nonenhancing, low-density, wedge-shaped defect retracts from the normally perfused renal parenchyma. In

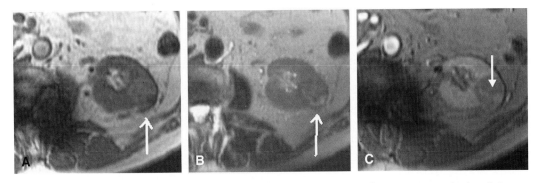

Fig. 15. Preoperative MRI of ultimately unsuccessful RFA. Tumor *demonstrates heterogeneous, predominantly intermediate SI on T1-WI (A—arrow) and on T2-WI (*B—arrow). Postcontrast T1-WI (*C*) demonstrates mild heterogeneous enhancement (*closed arrow*). (*From* Svatek RS, Sims R, Anderson JK, et al. Magnetic resonance imaging characteristics of renal tumors following radiofrequency ablation. Urology 2006;67(3):508–12; with permission.)

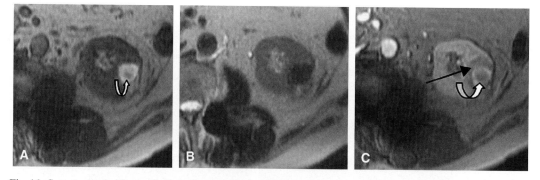

Fig. 16. Same tumor in Figure 15, six weeks postablation MRI. Ablation zone (*curved arrow*) characterized by high SI on T1-WI (*A*), low SI on T2-WI (*B*), and lack of enhancement on postcontrast T1-WI (*C*). Ablation zone does not occupy the region of tumor completely, suggesting incomplete ablation (*straight arrow*). (*From* Svatek RS, Sims R, Anderson JK, et al. Magnetic resonance imaging characteristics of renal tumors following radiofrequency ablation. Urology 2006;67(3):508–12; with permission.)

Matsumoto's CT series at 12 months four of eight (50%) endophytic tumors were separated from the normal renal tissue by a thin rim of fat (Fig. 13). Exophytic tumors displayed retraction from the renal parenchyma to a lesser extent. Gervais and colleagues made similar observations in their series of 23 RFA ablations [28].

Local recurrences following radiofrequency ablation

Local recurrence following RFA is infrequent. In most series, the definition of recurrence has been based on radiologic follow-up without pathologic confirmation and occurs in 0% to 15% of cases [27–29,34,38,39]. As most of these diagnoses were made before metastatic spread, radiographic surveillance permits identification and retreatment strategies. For example, in the one case in the authors' series, a patient underwent an uncomplicated percutaneous ablation of a 3.3 cm posterior endophytic tumor. After initial follow-up at 6 weeks, the patient was lost to follow-up until 24 months later, when a spherical centrally located area of enhancement was encountered adjacent to the ablation zone (Fig. 17). Laparoscopic nephrectomy was performed, and pathology revealed a clear cell renal cell carcinoma 3.2 cm in diameter within the ablation zone.

Because late local recurrences following RFA are uncommon, it is difficult to define the conclusive radiologic characteristics of a malignant recurrence. In the authors' opinion, however, a spherical area of enhancement, similar to a primary renal cell carcinoma, is particularly worrisome. Irregular nodularity at the periphery of the ablation zone in the perinephric fat (distinct from the ablated tumor) appears to be part of the normal granulomatous evolution following RFA for a small percentage of patients (Fig. 18). Undoubtedly, as imaging technology progresses and

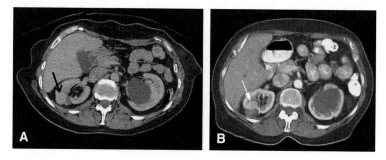

Fig. 17. CT scans of a right-sided renal tumor that had a subsequent late local recurrence following RFA. (*A*) Preablation image showing enhancing tumor (*black arrow*). Patient was then lost to follow-up until 24 months after ablation. (*B*) Scan 24 months after ablation showing spherical area of enhancement at the central edge of the tumor (*white arrow*). On nephrectomy, this tumor contained renal cell carcinoma.

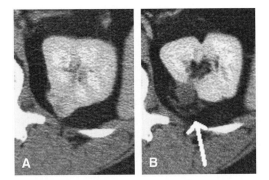

Fig. 18. Contrast enhanced CT scans of a posterior left-sided renal tumor that had subsequent nodular growth in the perinephric fat. (*A*) Preablation image. (*B*) Scan 12 months after ablation. There is a slight thickening in the peri-tumor halo (*arrow*) but no enhancement. Nodular thickening with enhancement may occur in the perinephric tissue, which occurred in this case. Nephrectomy demonstrated this nodular thickening contained only fat necrosis and a foreign body giant cell reaction. There was no evidence of malignancy.

experience with renal RFA grows, the diagnosis of a late malignant recurrence following RFA will be recognized with greater sensitivity and specificity.

Summary

As new minimally invasive treatment options for small renal tumors have been developed, the reliance upon imaging technologies intraoperatively and postoperatively has expanded. CT, MRI, and ultrasonography are useful adjuvants for intra- and postoperative care, yet it is clear that further improvements can be made. Whether it is the addition of contrast-enhancement for ultrasonography, the refinement of CT, MRI, and PET techniques for the follow-up of ablated masses, or the development of an entirely new technology to diagnosis possible recurrences, improvements in imaging during and following minimally invasive renal surgery will provide greatly improved care. Equally important, the urologist of the 21st century must be facile at interpreting and manipulating these technologies to appropriately care for renal tumor patients.

References

[1] Konnak JW, Grossman HB. Renal cell carcinoma as an incidental finding. J Urol 1985;134:1094–6.

[2] Janzen NK, Kim HL, Figlin RA, et al. Surveillance after radical or partial nephrectomy for localized renal cell carcinoma and management of recurrent disease. Urol Clin North Am 2003;30:843–52.

[3] Gill IS, Desai MM, Kaouk JH, et al. Laparoscopic partial nephrectomy for renal tumor: duplicating open surgical techniques. J Urol 2002;167:469–76 [discussion 475–6].

[4] Nguyen TT, Parkinson JP, Kuehn DM, et al. Technique for ensuring negative surgical margins during laparoscopic partial nephrectomy. J Endourol 2005;19:410–5.

[5] Gill IS, Matin SF, Desai MM, et al. Comparative analysis of laparoscopic versus open partial nephrectomy for renal tumors in 200 patients. J Urol 2003; 170:64–8.

[6] Link RE, Bhayani SB, Allaf ME, et al. Exploring the learning curve, pathological outcomes and perioperative morbidity of laparoscopic partial nephrectomy performed for renal mass. J Urol 2005; 173:1690–4.

[7] Gill IS, Hsu TH, Fox RL, et al. Laparoscopic and percutaneous radiofrequency ablation of the kidney: acute and chronic porcine study. Urology 2000;56: 197–200.

[8] Gervais DA, McGovern FJ, Wood BJ, et al. Radio-frequency ablation of renal cell carcinoma: early clinical experience. Radiology 2000;217: 665–72.

[9] Johnson DB, Duchene DA, Taylor GD, et al. Contrast-enhanced ultrasound evaluation of radiofrequency ablation of the kidney: reliable imaging of the thermolesion. J Endourol 2005;19:248–52.

[10] Slabaugh TK, Machaidze Z, Hennigar R, et al. Monitoring radiofrequency renal lesions in real time using contrast-enhanced ultrasonography: a porcine model. J Endourol 2005;19:579–83.

[11] Lewin JS, Nour SG, Connell CF, et al. Phase II clinical trial of interactive MR imaging-guided interstitial radiofrequency thermal ablation of primary kidney tumors: initial experience. Radiology 2004; 232:835–45.

[12] Remer EM, Weinberg EJ, Oto A, et al. MR imaging of the kidneys after laparoscopic cryoablation. AJR Am J Roentgenol 2000;174:635–40.

[13] Chen RN, Novick AC, Gill IS. Laparoscopic cryoablation of renal masses. Urol Clin North Am 2000; 27:813–20.

[14] Nadler RB, Kim SC, Rubenstein JN, et al. Laparoscopic renal cryosurgery: the Northwestern experience. J Urol 2003;170:1121–5.

[15] Cestari A, Guazzoni G, dell'Acqua V, et al. Laparoscopic cryoablation of solid renal masses: intermediate-term follow-up. J Urol 2004;172:1267–70.

[16] Dechet CB, Zincke H, Sebo TJ, et al. Prospective analysis of computerized tomography and needle biopsy with permanent sectioning to determine the nature of solid renal masses in adults. J Urol 2003;169: 71–4.

[17] Campbell SC, Novick AC, Herts B, et al. Prospective evaluation of fine needle aspiration of small, solid renal masses: accuracy and morbidity. Urology 1997; 50:25–9.

[18] Zhu Q, Shimizu T, Endo H, et al. Assessment of renal cell carcinoma after cryoablation using contrast-enhanced gray-scale ultrasound: a case series. Clin Imaging 2005;29:102–8.

[19] Gill IS, Novick AC, Meraney AM, et al. Laparoscopic renal cryoablation in 32 patients. Urology 2000;56:748–53.

[20] Rodriguez R, Chan DY, Bishoff JT, et al. Renal ablative cryosurgery in selected patients with peripheral renal masses. Urology 2000;55:25–30.

[21] Lee DI, McGinnis DE, Feld R, et al. Retroperitoneal laparoscopic cryoablation of small renal tumors: intermediate results. Urology 2003;61:83–8.

[22] Gupta A, Allaf ME, Kavoussi LR, et al. Percutaneous renal tumor cryoablation under CT guidance: Initial clinical experience. J Urol 2006;175:447–52.

[23] Shingleton WB, Farabaugh P, Hughson M, et al. Percutaneous cryoablation of porcine kidneys with magnetic resonance imaging monitoring. J Urol 2001;166:289–91.

[24] Dunnich N, Sandler C, Amis E, et al. Textbook of uroradiology. 2nd edition. Philadelphia (PA): Lippincott, Williams, and Wilkins; 1997.

[25] Pavlovich CP, Walther MM, Choyke PL, et al. Percutaneous radio frequency ablation of small renal tumors: initial results. J Urol 2002;167:10–5.

[26] Roy-Choudhury SH, Cast JE, Cooksey G, et al. Early experience with percutaneous radiofrequency ablation of small solid renal masses. AJR Am J Roentgenol 2003;180:1055–61.

[27] Mayo-Smith WW, Dupuy DE, Parikh PM, et al. Imaging-guided percutaneous radiofrequency ablation of solid renal masses: techniques and outcomes of 38 treatment sessions in 32 consecutive patients. AJR Am J Roentgenol 2003;180:1503–8.

[28] Gervais DA, McGovern FJ, Arellano RS, et al. Renal cell carcinoma: clinical experience and technical success with radio-frequency ablation of 42 tumors. Radiology 2003;226:417–24.

[29] Hwang JJ, Walther MM, Pautler SE, et al. Radio frequency ablation of small renal tumors:: intermediate results. J Urol 2004;171:1814–8.

[30] Matsumoto ED, Johnson DB, Ogan K, et al. Short-term efficacy of temperature-based radiofrequency ablation of small renal tumors. Urology 2005;65:877–81.

[31] Rendon RA, Gertner MR, Sherar MD, et al. Development of a radiofrequency based thermal therapy technique in an in vivo porcine model for the treatment of small renal masses. J Urol 2001;166:292–8.

[32] Marcovich R, Aldana JP, Morgenstern N, et al. Optimal lesion assessment following acute radio frequency ablation of porcine kidney: cellular viability or histopathology? J Urol 2003;170:1370–4.

[33] Svatek R, Sims R, Anderson JK, et al. Magnetic resonance imaging following radiofrequency ablation of renal tumors. Urology 2006;67:508–12.

[34] Matsumoto ED, Watumull L, Johnson DB, et al. The radiographic evolution of radio frequency ablated renal tumors. J Urol 2004;172:45–8.

[35] Pantuck AJ, Zisman A, Cohen J, et al. Cryosurgical ablation of renal tumors using 1.5 mm, ultrathin cryoprobes. Urology 2002;59:130–3.

[36] Zlotta AR, Wildschutz T, Raviv G, et al. Radiofrequency interstitial tumor ablation (RITA) is a possible new modality for treatment of renal cancer: ex vivo and in vivo experience. J Endourol 1997;11:251–8.

[37] Johnson DB, Saboorian MH, Duchene DA, et al. Nephrectomy after radiofrequency ablation-induced ureteropelvic junction obstruction: potential complication and long-term assessment of ablation adequacy. Urology 2003;62:351–2.

[38] Farrell MA, Charboneau WJ, DiMarco DS, et al. Imaging-guided radiofrequency ablation of solid renal tumors. AJR Am J Roentgenol 2003;180:1509–13.

[39] Su LM, Jarrett TW, Chan DY, et al. Percutaneous computed tomography-guided radiofrequency ablation of renal masses in high surgical risk patients: preliminary results. Urology 2003;61:26–33.

ELSEVIER
SAUNDERS

Urol Clin N Am 33 (2006) 353–364

UROLOGIC
CLINICS
of North America

Imaging for Percutaneous Renal Access and Management of Renal Calculi

Sangtae Park, MD, MPH[a], Margaret S. Pearle, MD, PhD[b],*

[a]University of Washington School of Medicine, Seattle, WA, USA
[b]The University of Texas Southwestern Medical Center, 5323 Harry Hines Boulevard,
Dallas, J8.106, TX 75390, USA

Choosing the optimal treatment modality for patients who have renal calculi depends on appropriate imaging studies that define the stone burden and renal anatomy and that delineate the anatomic relations of the kidney to surrounding organs. Percutaneous nephrostolithotomy (PCNL) is the treatment of choice for patients who have large or complex renal calculi and for those in whom shock wave lithotripsy (SWL) or ureteroscopy (URS) have failed. It is also an option for patients who have concurrent stones and ureteropelvic junction obstruction.

Radiographic imaging is an integral part of the planning and performing of percutaneous renal surgery. Preoperative imaging allows a priori selection of optimal percutaneous renal access. Intraoperative imaging is necessary to carry out directed percutaneous renal puncture and to facilitate endoscopic inspection. Finally, postoperative imaging ascertains the presence and location of residual calculi and determines the need for second-look flexible nephroscopy.

Knowledge of the indications for and selection of appropriate imaging studies for preoperative planning, intraoperative treatment, and postoperative assessment is essential for safe and efficacious percutaneous renal stone surgery.

Preoperative imaging

Pre-operative imaging studies define the renal or ureteral stone burden and delineate renal

anatomy and the relationship of the kidney to surrounding organs. Selecting the optimal preoperative imaging study depends on the patient's renal function, body habitus, and renal anatomy. Contrast studies may be unsafe in patients who have renal insufficiency, and consequently, detailed collecting of system anatomy may be unattainable except at the time of surgery. In patients who have renal anomalies such as horseshoe kidney, or with an unusual body habitus caused by severe scoliosis or meningomyelocele, the relationship of the kidney to surrounding organs that are potentially in the line of percutaneous puncture may be atypical, and consequently cross-sectional imaging studies are needed to determine a safe line of access.

Plain abdominal radiography

Most calcium-containing stones are visible on plain abdominal radiograph (KUB) provided they are sufficiently large, not obscured by overlying stool or bowel gas, and not overlying the spine or bony pelvis. Brushite and calcium oxalate monohydrate stones are the most radio-opaque of calcium-containing stones, followed by calcium apatite and calcium oxalate dihydrate stones. Cystine and struvite stones are faintly opaque, and uric acid stones are radiolucent, although they may be faintly visible when mixed with calcium, or when they reach a large size.

Although KUB has the advantage of being rapidly acquired, readily available, and relatively inexpensive, its use is limited by a fairly low sensitivity for the detection of renal calculi. Indeed, published sensitivity and specificity rates for

* Corresponding author.
E-mail address: margaret.pearle@utsouthwestern.edu (M.S. Pearle).

KUB in the detection of renal and ureteral calculi range from 58% to 62% and 67% to 69%, respectively [1–4]. Furthermore, the lack of anatomic detail with regard to the kidney and surrounding organs limits its usefulness in preoperative planning for PCNL. KUB, however, is useful in determining if a stone is radio-opaque and can be identified on fluoroscopy at the time of percutaneous renal access. For nonopaque stones, opacification of the renal collecting system with retrograde injection of contrast, or use of ultrasound guidance, may be necessary to obtain percutaneous access.

Intravenous urogram

Historically, the intravenous urogram (IVU) was the study of choice for evaluating patients with suspected stones and for planning therapy [5,6]. IVU demonstrates detailed collecting system anatomy, particularly when appropriate oblique and anteroposterior views are obtained. In addition, it shows the relation of the kidney and collecting system to the ribs, which determines the need for supracostal access. On the other hand, IVU typically is performed in the supine position, and the relation of the collecting system to the pleural space and ribs may change when the patient is prone. Nevertheless, the IVU can assist in selecting the appropriate calyx for percutaneous puncture based on the location of the stone, the infundibulopelvic angle, and the spatial anatomy of the collecting system. In many cases, direct access into the stone-bearing calyx is optimal. In other cases, such as a complete staghorn calculus, or a partial staghorn calculus occupying the renal pelvis and multiple lower pole calyces, an upper pole posterior calyx may serve as the site of optimal access (Fig. 1). IVU is important in planning the percutaneous approach to stone-bearing calyceal diverticula, as it delineates the calyx with which the diverticulum is associated and shows the size and location of the diverticulum (Fig. 2).

Because nonenhanced, helical CT is superior to IVU for detecting renal and ureteral calculi, IVU is no longer available at some institutions [7–11]. Nevertheless, the detailed depiction of collecting system anatomy with IVU remains an important adjunct in the evaluation of patients considered for PCNL. Whether CT urography with three-dimensional reconstruction will prove to be as good or superior to IVU and ultimately replace IVU for the delineation of collecting system anatomy remains to be seen [12–14].

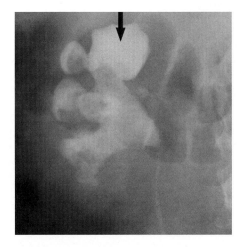

Fig. 1. Intravenous urogram demonstrates a staghorn calculus occupying most of the collecting system. The upper pole calyx (*arrow*) is the optimal site for percutaneous puncture to access all the branches of this stone.

CT

With the introduction of unenhanced helical CT, detection of renal and ureteral calculi has been enhanced greatly [7,9,15]. Indeed, CT has been shown to be superior to IVU for evaluating patients with acute flank pain [8,16–18]. In this clinical setting, the reported sensitivity and specificity of helical CT for ureteral calculi ranges from 94% to 100% and from 94% to 97%, respectively [9,10,16,18].

The benefits of CT imaging before PCNL, however, surpass just the accurate detection of renal calculi. CT delineates the extent, orientation, and location of renal calculi, which can facilitate the selection of an appropriate calyx for percutaneous access [12,14,19]. Furthermore, CT provides detailed information on the relational anatomy of the kidney that may impact selection of an appropriate calyx for safe puncture [20,21]. Knowledge of the relationship of the collecting system to adjacent organs such as colon, liver, or spleen helps avoid percutaneous puncture through these organs into the calyx of interest [22,23]. In addition, the proximity of the calyx to the pleural space generally can be ascertained by CT. Hopper and colleagues estimated the likelihood of lung injury from supracostal access by performing CT scans with sagittal reconstructions at maximal inspiration and expiration, and found that at end expiration, the likelihood of transgressing the pleura with a supracostal access was 29% on the right and 14% on the left [24].

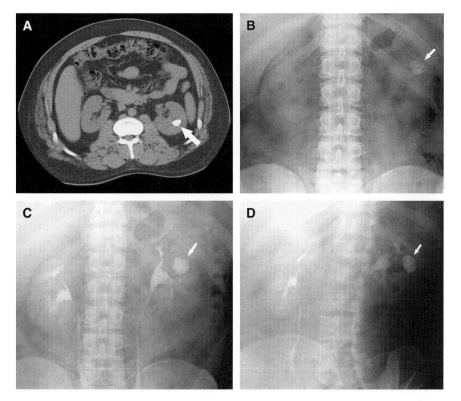

Fig. 2. (*A*) Noncontrast CT demonstrates a left renal calculus (*arrow*). (*B*) Scout film from intravenous urogram demonstrates that the left renal stone seen on CT is composed of multiple small stones (*arrow*). (*C*) Ten-minute film from intravenous urogram shows that the stones are located within a calyceal diverticulum (*arrow*). Noncontrast CT alone was not sufficient to reveal the caliceal diverticulum. (*D*) Oblique film shows that the stone-bearing diverticulum (*arrow*) projects posteriorly from the upper pole calyx.

Clinically, hydropneumothorax occurs in up to 12% of cases in which a supracostal access is used [25–32].

Some investigators, however, have questioned the applicability of CT performed in the supine position to percutaneous access that typically is performed in the prone position. Indeed, adjacent vital structures such as the colon, lung, and liver may move into the line of the puncture with a change in position. Sengupta and colleagues evaluated 14 patients undergoing supine CT, immediately followed by prone CT, and noted that the angle of the renal hilum relative to the vertebral column increased from 57° in the supine position to 62° in the prone position [33]. Although this difference was statistically significant, the authors observed that the relative orientation of the anterior and posterior calyces remained unchanged, and consequently they concluded that routine CT scanning in the supine position is sufficient for preoperative PCNL planning.

Ng and colleagues performed noncontrast, prone helical CT during inspiration and expiration, with three-dimensional reconstruction in six patients scheduled for PCNL [34]. In five of six patients, extrapleural percutaneous access at a favorable angle (perpendicular or directed caudally) was deemed possible, and both inspiratory and expiratory phase images were necessary to determine the optimal access site. In one patient with a stone-bearing calyceal diverticulum, a safe access site could not be identified, and the patient was treated laparoscopically. Simulated intercostal access during the inspiratory phase appeared to be transpleural in all six cases, suggesting that expiratory phase access may be safer. Although most investigators recommend obtaining percutaneous access while the patient is in expiration, the incidence of pleural transgression with this maneuver is variable. Kekre and colleagues reported a nearly 10% incidence of pleural complications among 102 patients undergoing PCNL by means of a supracostal puncture during full expiration [28]. Stening and Bourne, however, reported no cases of pleural transgression in 21 patients who underwent supracostal access in full inspiration [27]. The difference in outcomes in these series may be accounted for by differences in the laterality of the access; medial access was performed purposefully by Kekre and colleagues [28], while access corresponding to the lateral half of the rib was performed by Stening and Bourne [27]. Maheshwari and colleagues noted their experience in 150 patients undergoing PCNL at full expiration with no pleural complications, and concurred with Stening and Bourne on the importance of a lateral approach to supracostal puncture [35].

Enhanced computing power and sophisticated three-dimensional CT software have led to the capability of creating detailed three-dimensional CT urography images depicting the renal parenchyma and pyelocaliceal system (Fig. 3) [13,14]. With the use of three-dimensional CT imaging, the collecting system and its relational anatomy to adjacent structures can be viewed readily, and an optimal and safe access site selected. Initially, three-dimensional CT was used to produce surface-rendered models, but the time required for data acquisition was prohibitive, and reconstruction was unreliable [36]. Moreover, once contrast was administered, the stone was indistinguishable from the collecting system. Later, three-dimensional CT reconstruction of staghorn calculi was used to facilitate selection of the percutaneous puncture site for PCNL (Fig. 4) [14,19,37]. Investigators, however, differed in their perception of the value of these images over conventional IVU and CT for preoperative planning.

Recently, Ghani and colleagues used a 16-slice CT scanner to obtain 2.5 mm-thick slices through the kidney in a patient who had a stone in a horseshoe kidney [21]. Using noncontrast and contrast-enhanced images, a 360°, rotating volume-rendered movie of the collecting system was reconstructed in only 45 seconds. The authors noted that the three-dimensional images depicted pelvicaliceal anatomy clearly, and were consistent with the IVU. The authors played this three-dimensional movie on a personal computer in the operating room to assist in selecting a calyx for percutaneous access in this patient.

In patients with an unusual body habitus, such as patients with spina bifida or severe scoliosis, percutaneous puncture using standard intraoperative fluoroscopy may be unsafe because of inability to identify the adjacent bowel, pleura, liver, or spleen that may be more likely to be violated in these patients (Fig. 5). As such, CT-guided percutaneous access before planned PCNL may be advantageous. Matlaga and colleagues reported that 3% of patients in their series of 154 PCNLs performed at two institutions underwent CT-guided renal access because of retrorenal colon, severe vertebral deformity, or stones in a transplant

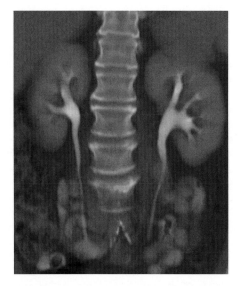

Fig. 3. CT urogram reconstructed with delayed contrast-enhanced images. The three-dimensional relationship of the collecting system to the ribs, pleura, and colon can be delineated.

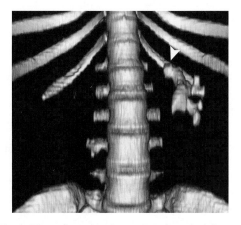

Fig. 4. Three-dimensional reconstruction of a left complete staghorn calculus. The superior border of the stone (*arrowhead*) lies just at the level of the 12th rib, and upper pole access likely would require a supracostal puncture.

In summary, preoperative imaging, primarily in the form of IVU or CT (either CT urogram or three-dimensional CT), is optimal to define the stone burden and to delineate the relational anatomy of the collecting system to surrounding organs and the pleural space. An appropriate calyx thus can be selected for safe percutaneous puncture that provides an optimal angle for access to the stone and entry into the collecting system.

Intraoperative imaging

Intraoperative imaging is necessary for obtaining percutaneous access, but it also facilitates endoscopic inspection of the collecting system. Percutaneous puncture can be guided by ultrasound or fluoroscopy. Although ultrasound guidance is sufficient for percutaneous puncture into the collecting system, passage of a guidewire and dilation of the tract requires the use of fluoroscopy.

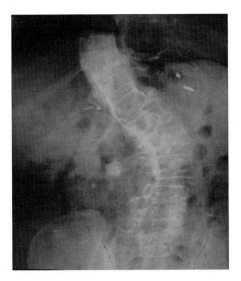

Fig. 5. Plain abdominal radiograph shows a large renal pelvic stone and a lower pole stone in a patient with severe kyphoscoliosis. Percutaneous access to the lower pole calyces could be difficult, as the kidney is displaced toward the iliac bone. In this setting, the distance between the 12th rib and the iliac bone can be very limited.

kidney [38]. After successful CT-guided access by the interventional radiologist, PCNL was completed safely by the urologist. Thus, in select cases, usually guided by findings on preoperative CT scan, CT-guided percutaneous access may be safer than traditional fluoroscopic-guided access. In these cases, the urologist should confer with the radiologist regarding selection of the appropriate calyx for percutaneous puncture.

Ultrasound

Ultrasound guidance can be used to direct percutaneous puncture into the collecting system. Limitations of this modality include limited targeting ability in a nondistended collecting system, poor image quality in an obese patient, and limited ability to identify fine details of collecting system anatomy, such as a calyx with a stenotic infundibulum. Ultrasound, however, is the modality of choice for percutaneous access in select patient populations, such as pregnant patients [39–42] or renal transplant patients [43,44], in whom fluoroscopy is contraindicated or ill-advised or when retrograde passage of a ureteral catheter for opacification of the collecting system is precluded. Among transplant patients, ultrasound guidance offers the advantage of identifying overlying bowel that must be avoided when puncturing the transplant kidney [44].

Although ultrasound is attractive because it minimizes exposure of the patient and surgeon to ionizing radiation, it is strongly operator-dependent. Furthermore, although large intrarenal stones and hydroureteronephrosis are readily evident, smaller stones and those in the ureter may be difficult to identify by ultrasound. In addition, ultrasound is unable to differentiate nephrocalcinosis from nephrolithiasis, mandating further imaging modalities.

MRI

MRI has assumed a very limited role in the diagnosis and management of renal calculi because of unreliable identification of stones in the collecting system or ureter. Because it avoids ionizing radiation, MRI may be considered an alternative to ultrasound in the pregnant patient with suspected stones, but the greater availability, lower cost, and greater accuracy of ultrasound in the diagnosis of stones and obstruction make MRI a rarely used modality. The use of open configuration MRI to facilitate percutaneous nephrostomy placement has been described, but this application is considered investigatory, and its future potential is unclear [39]. At the current time, MRI is not considered a first-line imaging modality for preoperative planning for PCNL.

Fluoroscopy

Fluoroscopy is the most common imaging modality used to obtain percutaneous renal access, although the choice between fluoroscopy and ultrasound is dependent on surgeon preference and experience. Regardless of the imaging modality used to gain access, intraoperative fluoroscopy is indispensable for the successful completion of PCNL.

To facilitate fluoroscopic-guided percutaneous puncture, dilute contrast or air is instilled by means of a retrograde ureteral catheter or occlusion balloon catheter placed cystoscopically at the time of PCNL. Opacification of the collecting system delineates and distends the collecting system, further facilitating access. The instillation of air to create an air pyelogram has an advantage over instilling contrast in that air can identify the posterior calyces and avoids obscuring the stone (Fig. 6). The location of the stone-bearing calyces and their relation to the overlying ribs allows the surgeon to target the appropriate calyx, taking into account the risk of pleural violation. Upper pole percutaneous puncture provides optimal access to large or complex renal calculi, to stones isolated in the upper pole calyces, to lower pole partial staghorn calculi, and to large ureteropelvic junction stones [30]. Lower pole access is favored for a primarily lower pole stone burden or for renal pelvic stones. Midpole access generally is reserved for direct puncture onto isolated midpole stones, because access into these calyces may not allow inspection of either the upper or lower pole calyces.

After debulking the stone with rigid nephroscopy, flexible nephroscopy is performed to inspect the entire collecting system and to retrieve stones remote from the nephrostomy tract that are not accessible with the rigid nephroscope. Entry into each calyx is documented fluoroscopically by injecting dilute contrast through the nephroscope when each calyx is entered (Fig. 7). Likewise, the ureter must be endoscopically or radiographically cleared by direct endoscopic inspection or by injection of contrast through the nephroscope down the ureter. Correct nephrostomy tube placement also is ensured with intraoperative antegrade nephrostogram.

The introduction of CT fluoroscopy, whereby live CT can be performed in the operating room, has the potential to allow percutaneous access to be performed under CT guidance with real-time visualization. CT fluoroscopy also has the potential to allow more accurate detection of residual fragments intraoperatively, thereby precluding the need for second-look flexible nephroscopy. Although CT fluoroscopy has not reached widespread use, and there are no reports of intraoperative use for PCNL, application of this modality to percutaneous brachytherapy for rectal cancer [45] and radiofrequency ablation of pulmonary masses has been reported [46].

The last step of PCNL is fluoroscopic inspection of the chest to assess for hydrothorax. Supracostal percutaneous puncture (above the 12th rib) is associated with a 0% to 12% incidence of pleural complications [25–32]. The risk of hydropneumothorax with access above the 11th rib approaches 35% [30]. Intraoperative chest fluoroscopy has the advantage of reliably identifying pleural fluid that can be drained intraoperatively, while the patient is anesthetized (Fig. 8). Because the fluid usually is composed primarily of irrigant, placement of a small bore (8 to 10 F) thoracostomy tube is generally sufficient for drainage, and can be placed with the same equipment and technique used to obtain percutaneous access (see Fig. 8). Ogan and colleagues compared the sensitivity of intraoperative chest fluoroscopy with immediate postoperative recovery room chest radiograph and postoperative day 1 CT of the kidneys and lung bases in 89 consecutive patients undergoing PCNL [47]. Among this group, 58% of patients underwent supracostal puncture, and seven patients required tube thoracostomy for hydropneumothorax, two of whom were detected

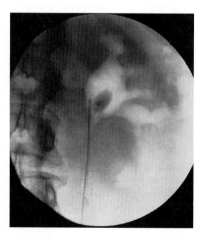

Fig. 6. Air pyelogram obtained by retrograde instillation of air through an externalized ureteral catheter. In the prone position, posterior calyces preferentially become air-filled.

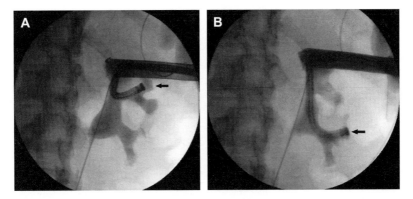

Fig. 7. (*A,B*) Flexible nephroscopy with opacification of calyces as they are entered to document and confirm entry into each calyx (*arrows*).

by intraoperative chest fluoroscopy. The other cases were diagnosed postoperatively when the patients developed symptoms. In no case, was intervention initiated on the basis of immediate postoperative chest radiograph when intraoperative fluoroscopy was negative, suggesting that intraoperative fluoroscopy is sufficient to assess the chest after PCNL. Patient symptoms should prompt chest imaging postoperatively. Thus, routine postoperative chest radiography is neither necessary nor cost-effective in patients who have been evaluated by intraoperative fluoroscopy.

Radiation safety

Although the urologist can limit radiation exposure to the patient outside the operating room by the judicious selection of pre- and postoperative imaging studies, intraoperative radiograph use falls under the direct control of the surgeon and impacts not only patient but surgeon safety also. Because of the widespread use of ionizing radiation for medical diagnostic and therapeutic purposes, many states have established boards of radiological health and safety. In California for example, physicians using fluoroscopy are legally mandated to be licensed radiograph supervisors and operators, a process which requires completion of a computer-based examination on the principles of radiation physics and safety. The key principle in maximizing safety is to keep the exposure as low as reasonably achievable (ALARA), to protect the patient, physician, and other operating room personnel.

Knowledge of the quantity of radiation incurred during PCNL is critical to instituting means to minimize exposure. Hellawell and

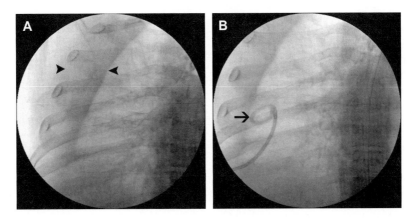

Fig. 8. (*A*) Fluoroscopic inspection of the chest after PCNL with supracostal access. Arrows depict a moderate-sized hydrothorax between the costal margin and lung parenchyma. (*B*) Successful placement of small bore thoracostomy tube (*arrow*) into the pleural space under fluoroscopic guidance.

colleagues measured radiation exposure during 18 ureteroscopy and six PCNL procedures during a 4-month period by placing thermoluminescent dosimeters in seven locations on the surgeon's body, including the forehead, the fifth digits of both hands, and both anterior legs and ankles [48]. During PCNL in which the radiograph tube of the C arm was placed under the patient and the image intensifier on top, as is routine, the greatest exposure from scattered radiation was recorded in the lower extremities, and the lowest exposure was recorded at eye level as recorded by the forehead dosimeter. Average fluoroscopy time was 10.7 minutes for PCNL. At a distance of 75 cm from the patient, a surgeon performing 50 PCNLs a year would receive a total body exposure of 2 to 8.4 mGy, with the lower value representing the ocular dose and the higher value occurring at the level of the legs. These doses represent 0.5% to 1.7% of the established allowable dose limit for radiation exposure in Great Britain [48].

Although this report suggests that radiation exposure to the surgeon is low, Yang and colleagues studied the use of a novel radiation shield during PCNL to further protect the surgeon from radiation exposure [49]. Using a 0.5 mm lead-equivalent vinyl-coated sheeting fastened to the operating table during PCNL, they demonstrated a 71% to 96% decrease in exposure to ionizing radiation using dosimeters.

Because the harmful effects of radiation do not occur at a threshold level, but rather in a dose-dependent manner, it is critical for the surgeon to understand basic radiation physics and to use the ALARA principle when performing PCNL. Exposure to primary radiation and scatter radiation should be minimized to protect the surgeon and patient. Scatter radiation occurs when the primary beam intercepts an object, typically the patient, and scatters x-rays. Scatter radiation is greatest below the operating table when the C arm is oriented with the image intensifier above the patient. In this orientation of the C arm, most of the scatter radiation is absorbed by the floor.

All personnel should wear safety lead aprons and stand as far away as possible from the radiograph source. Ambient light in the operating room should be minimized to provide optimal visibility of the fluoroscopic monitor. The surgeon should keep his/her hands out of the radiation field as much as possible. The use of lead gloves will reduce exposure of the hands to radiation during percutaneous puncture or during endoscopic inspection under fluoroscopic guidance. In addition, collimating the radiation beam to the area of interest and placing the image intensifier as close to the patient as possible reduces the exposure of the surgeon and patient to scatter radiation and avoids exposure of areas of the patient adjacent to the area of interest. Lastly, the pulsed fluoroscopy mode should be used whenever possible to minimize fluoroscopy on time [50].

Postoperative imaging

Post-PCNL imaging is aimed at identifying residual stones and establishing adequate antegrade drainage from the collecting system.

Plain abdominal radiographs and nephrotomograms

Traditionally, KUB or plain nephrotomograms were used to identify residual stones post-PCNL and determine the need for second-look flexible nephroscopy. Although these modalities are inexpensive and quick, their sensitivity in detecting residual calculi is marginal. Denstedt and colleagues compared the sensitivity of KUB and plain nephrotomograms in detecting residual calculi in 29 patients with large renal calculi undergoing PCNL [51]. Using second-look flexible nephroscopy as the gold standard for identifying residual stones, they found that KUB and nephrotomograms overestimated stone-free rates by 35% and 17%, respectively. Consequently, they encouraged the liberal use of flexible nephroscopy to achieve a stone-free state after PCNL, regardless of the results of the imaging studies.

CT

With the widespread use of nonenhanced helical CT to identify renal and ureteral calculi, recent investigators compared the sensitivity of noncontrast CT with flexible nephroscopy in detecting residual stones after PCNL. Pearle and colleagues prospectively compared KUB, noncontrast CT, and flexible nephroscopy for their ability to detect residual stones in 36 patients with 41 renal units undergoing PCNL for large or complex renal calculi [52]. Using flexible nephroscopy as the gold standard reference, CT had a sensitivity of 100% and specificity of 62%, compared with 46% and 82%, respectively, for KUB. Thus, in their series, selective use of flexible nephroscopy based on CT findings would have resulted in only 12% of patients undergoing an unnecessary operation compared with 32% of patients if flexible nephroscopy was performed in all patients, as was their routine. Furthermore, by eliminating an unnecessary procedure in 20% of patients, a cost savings of over $100,000 per 100 patients potentially could be realized.

Waldmann and colleagues also routinely performed post-PCNL CT and found no residual stones in 59% of 121 patients [53]. Patients with significant residual stones were treated with shock wave lithotripsy or second-look nephroscopy (35%), and the remaining patients were left untreated. Although not all patients subsequently underwent flexible nephroscopy in this retrospective series, the authors concluded that CT is far superior to plain renal nephrotomography in determining the need for a second-look procedure.

Along with accurate identification of residual stones, CT has the additional advantage of precisely pinpointing the location of residual fragments and their relation to the nephrostomy tract, further facilitating retrieval of residual stones (Fig. 9).

Although the superiority of CT over plain radiographs in detecting renal calculi is undisputed, the optimal CT parameters to detect calculi have not been established. With multi-detector CT scans, the thickness of the CT slice impacts the sensitivity and specificity in detecting calculi. With CT parameters adjusted to keep radiation exposure within an acceptable range, thinner slices lead to decreased signal-to-noise ratio. To determine the optimal setting to maximize sensitivity without undue noise and maintain an acceptable

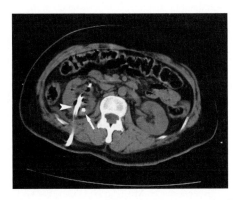

Fig. 9. Nonenhanced, helical CT obtained on the first postoperative day after PCNL demonstrates a solitary residual stone fragment (*arrow*) medial to nephrostomy tube (*arrowhead*).

radiation level, Memarsadeghi and colleagues randomized 147 patients with suspected stones to noncontrast CT imaging at 1.5 mm, 3 mm, and 5 mm slice thickness [11]. At a set dose of 11.4 mGy, total radiation, sensitivity and specificity were equivalent at 1.5 mm and 3 mm slices, but 5 mm slices led to a significantly higher frequency of missed stones. In this group, however, all 32 missed stones were less than 3 mm in size. Although the size cut-off for clinically insignificant residual stones has never been established, use of 3 mm slice thickness for CT imaging to detect residual calculi is advisable.

Although the sensitivity of CT in detecting renal calculi is unsurpassed, the reliability of CT in determining stone size has been questioned. Narepalem and colleagues compared size measurements of 58 stones on KUB and helical CT [54]. Although the measured transverse dimension was similar with the two modalities, CT tended to overestimate the cranio–caudal dimension of the stones by an average of 0.8 mm. In a similar study, Van Appledorn and colleagues concluded that helical CT overestimated stone size by 30% to 50% in the cranio–caudal dimension, compared with KUB [55]. In that study, the number of consecutive images in which a ureteral stone was visible on CT was multiplied by the reconstruction interval of 5 mm to create a size estimate, which was compared with the measurements of the same stone seen on the KUB film.

On the other hand, Kampa and colleagues reported that both urologists and radiologists routinely use "guestimations" when measuring stone size rather than actual measurements [56]. In their survey of 425 radiologists and urologists, a standard 11 mm stone was on average underestimated at 9.6 mm ($P<.02$), and up to 59% of practitioners admitted to using estimates rather than relying on electronic rulers for digital images.

Despite potential inaccuracies in measuring stone size, however, CT remains the best modality for detecting residual stones. The need for flexible nephroscopy based on the size of the residual fragments remains at the discretion of the surgeon.

Antegrade nephrostogram

Because of the potential for edema of the ureter or ureteropelvic junction as a result of previous stone or ureteral manipulation, antegrade nephrostogram is performed after most PCNL procedures to assure adequate antegrade drainage (Fig. 10). In addition, opacification of the collecting system can delineate calyceal anatomy, and along with noncontrast CT imaging, precisely localize residual stone fragments, thereby facilitating second-look flexible nephroscopy. If antegrade drainage is confirmed, the nephrostomy tube can be removed safely.

Summary

PCNL is an image-driven treatment modality that relies heavily on:

- Preoperative imaging to define stone burden and delineate the relational anatomy of the kidney
- Intraoperative imaging to facilitate percutaneous puncture, endoscopic inspection, and pleural screening
- Post-operative imaging to detect residual stones and assure antegrade drainage

The emergence of CT as the imaging modality of choice for detecting renal calculi and the ability of CT urography with or without three-dimensional reconstruction to delineate the collecting system make this the most versatile and sensitive imaging modality for use in PCNL. Fluoroscopy remains the mainstay of intraoperative imaging, but CT fluoroscopy holds promise in enhancing the ability to obtain safe percutaneous access and to detect residual stones. At present, IVU and ultrasound continue to play a role in the percutaneous management of patients who have renal calculi.

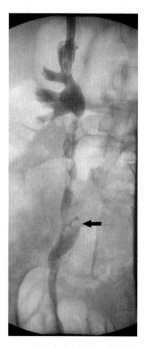

Fig. 10. Antegrade nephrostogram after PCNL shows filling of the collecting system and ureter and flow of contrast into the bladder. Filling defects in the ureter represent air bubbles (*arrow*). The nephrostomy tube can be removed safely.

References

[1] Roth CS, Bowyer BA, Berquist TH. Utility of the plain abdominal radiograph for diagnosing ureteral calculi. Ann Emerg Med 1985;14:311.

[2] Mutgi A, Williams JW, Nettleman M. Renal colic. Utility of the plain abdominal roentgenogram. Arch Intern Med 1991;151:1589.

[3] Jackman SV, Potter SR, Regan F, et al. Plain abdominal x-ray versus computerized tomography screening: sensitivity for stone localization after non-enhanced spiral computerized tomography. J Urol 2000;164:308.

[4] Boyd R, Gray AJ. Role of the plain radiograph and urinalysis in acute ureteric colic. J Accid Emerg Med 1996;13:390.

[5] Weiss A, Price R, Sage M, Barratt L. The intravenous pyelogram in renal colic. Australas Radiol 1988;32:429.

[6] Mutazindwa T, Husseini T. Imaging in acute renal colic: the intravenous urogram remains the gold standard. Eur J Radiol 1996;23:238.

[7] Sheley RC, Semonsen KG, Quinn SF. Helical CT in the evaluation of renal colic. Am J Emerg Med 1999; 17:279.

[8] Miller OF, Rineer SK, Reichard SR, et al. Prospective comparison of unenhanced spiral computed tomography and intravenous urogram in the evaluation of acute flank pain. Urology 1998;52:982.

[9] Boulay I, Holtz P, Foley WD, et al. Ureteral calculi: diagnostic efficacy of helical CT and implications for treatment of patients. AJR Am J Roentgenol 1999; 172:1485.

[10] Chen MY, Zagoria RJ. Can noncontrast helical computed tomography replace intravenous urography for evaluation of patients with acute urinary tract colic? J Emerg Med 1999;17:299.

[11] Memarsadeghi M, Heinz-Peer G, Helbich TH, et al. Unenhanced multi-detector row CT in patients suspected of having urinary stone disease: effect of section width on diagnosis. Radiology 2005;235:530.

[12] Thiruchelvam N, Mostafid H, Ubhayakar G. Planning percutaneous nephrolithotomy using multidetector computed tomography urography, multi-planar reconstruction and three-dimensional reformatting. BJU Int 2005;95:1280.

[13] Leder RA, Nelson RC. Three-dimensional CT of the genitourinary tract. J Endourol 2001;15:37.

[14] Buchholz NP. Three-dimensional CT scan stone reconstruction for the planning of percutaneous surgery in a morbidly obese patient. Urol Int 2000; 65:46.

[15] Heidenreich A, Desgrandschamps F, Terrier F. Modern approach of diagnosis and management of acute flank pain: review of all imaging modalities. Eur Urol 2002;41:351.

[16] Pfister SA, Deckart A, Laschke S, et al. Unenhanced helical computed tomography vs intravenous urography in patients with acute flank pain: accuracy and economic impact in a randomized prospective trial. Eur Radiol 2003;13:2513.

[17] Fielding JR, Steele G, Fox LA, et al. Spiral computerized tomography in the evaluation of acute flank pain: a replacement for excretory urography. J Urol 1997;157:2071.

[18] Yilmaz S, Sindel T, Arslan G, et al. Renal colic: comparison of spiral CT, US and IVU in the detection of ureteral calculi. Eur Radiol 1998;8:212.

[19] Hubert J, Blum A, Cormier L, et al. Three-dimensional CT-scan reconstruction of renal calculi. A new tool for mapping-out staghorn calculi and follow-up of radiolucent stones. Eur Urol 1997;31:297.

[20] Raj GV, Auge BK, Weizer AZ, et al. Percutaneous management of calculi within horseshoe kidneys. J Urol 2003;170:48.

[21] Ghani KR, Rintoul M, Patel U, et al. Three-dimensional planning of percutaneous renal stone surgery in a horseshoe kidney using 16-slice CT and volume-rendered movies. J Endourol 2005;19:461.

[22] Skoog SJ, Reed MD, Gaudier FA Jr, et al. The posterolateral and the retrorenal colon: implication in percutaneous stone extraction. J Urol 1985;134:110.

[23] Vallancien G, Capdeville R, Veillon B, et al. Colonic perforation during percutaneous nephrolithotomy. J Urol 1985;134:1185.

[24] Hopper KD, Yakes WF. The posterior intercostal approach for percutaneous renal procedures: risk of puncturing the lung, spleen, and liver as determined by CT. AJR Am J Roentgenol 1990;154:115.

[25] Young AT, Hunter DW, Castaneda-Zuniga WR, et al. Percutaneous extraction of urinary calculi: use of the intercostal approach. Radiology 1985; 154:633.

[26] Golijanin D, Katz R, Verstandig A, et al. The supracostal percutaneous nephrostomy for treatment of staghorn and complex kidney stones. J Endourol 1998;12:403.

[27] Stening SG, Bourne S. Supracostal percutaneous nephrolithotomy for upper pole caliceal calculi. J Endourol 1998;12:359.

[28] Kekre NS, Gopalakrishnan GG, Gupta GG, et al. Supracostal approach in percutaneous nephrolithotomy: experience with 102 cases. J Endourol 2001;15:789.

[29] Aron M, Goel R, Kesarwani PK, et al. Upper pole access for complex lower pole renal calculi. BJU Int 2004;94:849.

[30] Munver R, Delvecchio FC, Newman GE, et al. Critical analysis of supracostal access for percutaneous renal surgery. J Urol 2001;166:1242.

[31] Picus D, Weyman PJ, Clayman RV, et al. Intercostal space nephrostomy for percutaneous stone removal. AJR Am J Roentgenol 1986;147:393.

[32] Forsyth MJ, Fuchs EF. The supracostal approach for percutaneous nephrostolithotomy. J Urol 1987; 137:197.

[33] Sengupta S, Donnellan S, Vincent JM, et al. CT analysis of caliceal anatomy in the supine and prone positions. J Endourol 2000;14:555.

[34] Ng CS, Herts BR, Streem SB. Percutaneous access to upper pole renal stones: role of prone 3-dimensional computerized tomography in inspiratory and expiratory phases. J Urol 2005;173:124.

[35] Maheshwari PN, Chopade DK, Andankar MG. Comment on "supracostal approach in percutaneous nephrolithotomy: experience of 102 cases". J Endourol 2003;17:529.

[36] Heyns CF, van Gelderen WF. 3-dimensional imaging of the pelviocaliceal system by computerized tomographic reconstruction. J Urol 1990;144:1335.

[37] Liberman SN, Halpern EJ, Sullivan K, et al. Spiral computed tomography for staghorn calculi. Urology 1997;50:519.

[38] Matlaga BR, Shah OD, Zagoria RJ, et al. Computerized tomography guided access for percutaneous nephrostolithotomy. J Urol 2003;170:45.

[39] Evans HJ, Wollin TA. The management of urinary calculi in pregnancy. Curr Opin Urol 2001;11:379.

[40] McAleer SJ, Loughlin KR. Nephrolithiasis and pregnancy. Curr Opin Urol 2004;14:123.

[41] Kavoussi LR, Albala DM, Basler JW, et al. Percutaneous management of urolithiasis during pregnancy. J Urol 1992;148:1069.

[42] Fabrizio MD, Gray DS, Feld RI, et al. Placement of ureteral stents in pregnancy using ultrasound guidance. Tech Urol 1996;2:121.

[43] Francesca F, Felipetto R, Mosca F, et al. Percutaneous nephrolithotomy of transplanted kidney. J Endourol 2002;16:225.

[44] Lu HF, Shekarriz B, Stoller ML. Donor-gifted allograft urolithiasis: early percutaneous management. Urology 2002;59:25.

[45] Sakurai H, Mitsuhashi N, Harashima K, et al. CT-fluoroscopy guided interstitial brachytherapy with image-based treatment planning for unresectable locally recurrent rectal carcinoma. Brachytherapy 2004;3:222.

[46] Froelich JJ, Wagner HJ. CT-fluoroscopy: tool or gimmick? Cardiovasc Intervent Radiol 2001;24:297.

[47] Ogan K, Corwin TS, Smith T, et al. Sensitivity of chest fluoroscopy compared with chest CT and chest radiography for diagnosing hydropneumothorax in

association with percutaneous nephrostolithotomy. Urology 2003;62:988.

[48] Hellawell GO, Mutch SJ, Thevendran G, et al. Radiation exposure and the urologist: what are the risks? J Urol 2005;174:948.

[49] Yang RM, Morgan T, Bellman GC. Radiation protection during percutaneous nephrolithotomy: a new urologic surgery radiation shield. J Endourol 2002; 16:727.

[50] Norris TG. Radiation safety in fluoroscopy. Radiol Technol 2002;73:511.

[51] Denstedt JD, Clayman RV, Picus DD. Comparison of endoscopic and radiological residual fragment rate following percutaneous nephrolithotripsy. J Urol 1991;145:703.

[52] Pearle MS, Watamull LM, Mullican MA. Sensitivity of noncontrast helical computerized tomography and plain film radiography compared to flexible nephroscopy for detecting residual fragments after percutaneous nephrostolithotomy. J Urol 1999; 162:23.

[53] Waldmann TB, Lashley DB, Fuchs EF. Unenhanced computerized axial tomography to detect retained calculi after percutaneous ultrasonic lithotripsy. J Urol 1999;162:312.

[54] Narepalem N, Sundaram CP, Boridy IC, et al. Comparison of helical computerized tomography and plain radiography for estimating urinary stone size. J Urol 2002;167:1235.

[55] Van Appledorn S, Ball AJ, Patel VR, et al. Limitations of noncontrast CT for measuring ureteral stones. J Endourol 2003;17:851.

[56] Kampa RJ, Ghani KR, Wahed S, et al. Size Matters: A Survey of How Urinary-Tract Stones are Measured in the UK. J Endourol 2005;19: 856.

ELSEVIER
SAUNDERS

Urol Clin N Am 33 (2006) 365–376

UROLOGIC
CLINICS
of North America

Current Recommendations for Imaging in the Management of Urologic Traumas

Jason T. Jankowski, MD, J. Patrick Spirnak, MD*

Department of Urology, Case Western Reserve University, MetroHealth Medical Center, 2500 MetroHealth Drive, Room H947, Cleveland, OH 44109, USA

Trauma is the leading cause of death in young Americans. About 3% to 10% of patients who experience traumatic injuries will have involvement of the genitourinary tract [1,2]. Of these, the most commonly involved organ is the kidney, followed by the bladder, urethra, and ureter [2]. While much of the initial evaluation and resuscitation will be performed by an emergency room physician and trauma surgeon, it is important for a urologist to have early involvement and a clear understanding of both the mechanism and extent of injury. While the vast majority of traumatic urologic injuries are not life threatening, failure of diagnosis and delay in treatment can lead to significant patient morbidity.

The genitourinary tract has an amazing ability to heal itself. If the flow of urine can be maintained without obstruction, then healing of the traumatic injury is likely. The goal of the urologist in a trauma situation is thus threefold: (1) minimize hemorrhage, (2) maintain urinary flow without obstruction to preserve renal function, and (3) prevent extravasation of urine outside the urinary tract thereby decreasing the risk of local and systemic infection. With these goals in mind, proper imaging to correctly identify urologic injuries becomes of paramount importance. This paper will review the most current imaging modalities available to the practicing urologist. It will also define the clinical indications for each of these modalities.

* Corresponding author.
E-mail address: pspirnak@metrohealth.org
(J.P. Spirnak).

Renal trauma

The kidney is clearly the most commonly injured urologic organ. About 85% to 95% of these injuries are due to blunt trauma, with the remainder a result of penetrating injuries [3,4]. In recent decades, rapid access to precise radiographic imaging has led to a significant shift in the management of renal trauma. The vast majority of these injuries, both blunt and penetrating, are now managed nonoperatively.

Indications for renal imaging

Specific imaging criteria have been developed to identify those trauma victims who are likely to have major renal injuries. Radiographic imaging is recommended in all adult blunt trauma patients who present with either gross hematuria or hypotension (defined as a systolic blood pressure of less then 90 mm Hg at any time during resuscitation/evaluation). This recommendation is based on data that show about 12.5% of patients with either of these symptoms will have a major renal injury [5]. Only 0.2% of adult blunt trauma patients who present with microhematuria and a systolic blood pressure above 90 mm Hg will have a significant renal injury. This was validated by a prospective study that demonstrated that these patients can be followed clinically without radiographic imaging [5]. Despite the above criteria, one should obtain radiographic imaging if the history or examination is suggestive of renal injury: a rapid deceleration injury (high-speed motor vehicle accidents, fall from heights), flank ecchymosis, rib fractures, or lumbar spine or transverse process fractures.

Traditionally, all pediatric blunt trauma patients with any degree of hematuria have undergone radiographic imaging. Previous studies have shown that children are at greater risk of renal trauma after blunt abdominal injury when compared with adults [6]. Recent studies have suggested adopting criteria similar to that of adult patients to determine who requires radiographic assessment [7]. This clinical situation will remain controversial until a prospective study is performed.

All penetrating trauma patients require radiographic imaging if clinically stable. The degree of hematuria, presence of hypotension, and location of entry are not reliable in determining which patients require radiographic imaging.

Radiographic assessment

Computerized tomography

The gold standard for imaging renal injuries is contrast-enhanced computerized tomography (CT). Rapid spiral scanners are now readily available at most trauma centers and allow for thin-cut, high-quality images to be obtained in a matter of minutes. Contrast-enhanced CT allows for clear delineation of parenchymal lesions, identification of associated hematomas, and detection of urine extravasation. In addition, associated solid-organ injuries can be identified.

It is crucial that after initial scanning of the abdomen and pelvis is completed, a second scan—approximately 10 minutes after contrast injection—is performed to fully evaluate the collecting system. Studies at our institution have shown that without obtaining a delayed scan, 8.6% of collecting system injuries were missed [8].

The American Association for the Surgery of Trauma has developed a classification system for renal injuries based on depth of injury, vascular involvement, and presence of urinary extravasation [9] (see Box 1, Fig. 1).

The majority of renal injuries seen are classified as grade 1 (see Fig. 2). Renal contusions are seen as either ill defined or sharply defined areas of hypoenhancement. Subcapsular hematomas present as high-density fluid collections between the renal capsule and parenchyma. They frequently compress the underlying parenchyma, leading to a deformity in shape.

Nonexpanding perinephric hematomas are classified as grade 2 injuries (see Fig. 3). They appear on CT as high-density, ill-defined collections between Gerota's fascia and the renal parenchyma. They can be quite large, but typically do not cause deformity of the kidney.

Box 1. American Association for the Surgery of Trauma Classification System for Renal Injuries

Grade 1 injuries
- hematuria with normal imaging
- contusions
- subcapsular, nonexpanding hematoma without parenchymal laceration

Grade 2 injuries
- nonexpanding perinephric hematomas confined to the retroperitoneum
- renal cortical lacerations less than 1 cm in depth without urinary extravasation

Grade 3 injuries
- renal cortical lacerations greater than 1 cm in depth without urinary extravasation

Grade 4 injuries
- parenchymal laceration extending through renal cortex/medulla and into collecting system
- main renal artery or vein injury with contained hemorrhage
- segmental infarction without associated laceration

Grade 5 injuries
- shattered or devascularized kidney
- complete avulsion or thrombosis of mail renal artery or vein
- Ureteropelvic junction avulsion

Renal lacerations manifest as irregular, low-attenuation defects in the renal parenchyma. There is often an associated perinephric fluid collection. Lacerations are graded 2 to 4 based on depth and whether there is urinary extravasation (see Figs. 3 and 4). Delayed images are necessary to identify urinary extravasation. A "shattered kidney," or grade 5 parencymal injury, suggests multiple parencymal lacerations (see Fig. 5). There are often associated areas of infarction and urinary extravasation.

Segmental infarctions are also classified as grade 4 injuries (see Fig. 6). They appear as well-circumscribed areas of nonenhancement within the parenchyma and are a result of either thrombosis or laceration of segmental arteries.

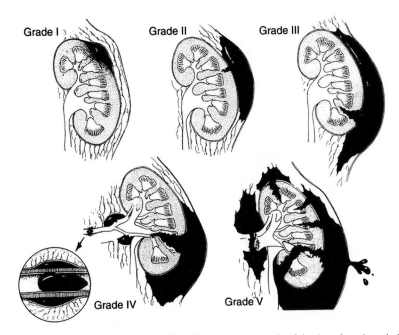

Fig. 1. Classification of renal injuries by grade, based on the organ injury scale of the American Association for the Surgery of Trauma. (*From* McAninch JW, Santucci RA. Genitourinary trauma. In: Walsh PC, Retik AB, Vaughan ED, et al, editors. Campbell's urology. 8th edition. Philadelphia: WB Saunders; 2002. p. 3709.)

Vascular injuries are classified as either grade 4 or 5. Bright enhancement of similar density to nearby vessel during initial phases of scanning suggests hemorrhage. A contained hemorrhage, also termed pseudoaneurysm, is usually well circumscribed (see Fig. 7). Active hemorrhage is usually more ill defined and there is often layering of contrast in the associated hematoma (see Fig. 8). A devascularized kidney will show no enhancement (see Fig. 9).

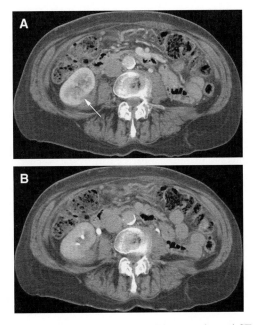

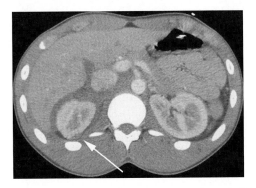

Fig. 2. Grade 1 renal injury. Contrast-enhanced CT scan of a patient involved in a motor vehicle accident demonstrates a small area of hypoenhancement along the posterior aspect of the right kidney (*arrow*).

Fig. 3. Grade 2 renal injury. (*A*) Contrast-enhanced CT scan of a patient who fell from a ladder demonstrates a low-attenuation defect in the posterior right renal cortex (*arrow*) with an associated perinephric hematoma. (*B*) Delayed image does not reveal urinary extravasation.

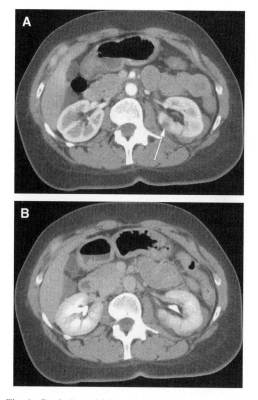

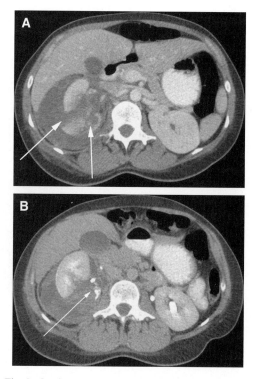

Fig. 4. Grade 3 renal injury. (*A*) Contrast-enhanced CT scan of a patient involved in a motorcycle accident reveals a low-attenuation defect in the medial left renal parenchyma (*arrow*) extending greater than 1cm into the cortex. (*B*) Delayed image does not reveal urinary extravasation.

Fig. 5. Grade 5 renal injury: shattered kidney. (*A*) Contrast-enhanced CT of a patient involved in a high-speed motor vehicle accident demonstrates multiple deep hypodense lacerations extending through renal parenchyma with a large perirenal hematoma (*arrows*). (*B*) Delayed image from same CT demonstrates urinary extravasation (*arrow*).

Ureteropelvic avulsion is classified as a grade 5 injury (see Fig. 10). There is extravasation of urine seen on delayed images. Complete avulsion can be differentiated from a partial tear by the absence of contrast in the distal ureter.

Other imaging modalities

In the United States, ultrasonography (US) has been popularized as a means to evaluate blunt abdominal trauma patients. This usually consists of a focused abdominal sonogram, commonly referred to as a FAST scan (Focused Assessment Sonography for Trauma). Typically, six specific areas are examined for the presence of free fluid: (1) the pericardial space, (2) the hepatorenal recess, (3) the splenorenal recess, (4,5) the right and left paracolic gutters, and (6) the pelvis [10]. The scan is usually performed by an emergency room physician or trauma surgeon in the trauma bay as resuscitation commences. While FAST

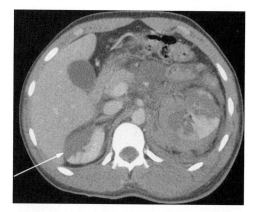

Fig. 6. Grade 4 renal injury: segmental infarct. Contrast-enhanced CT from a patient involved in a high-speed motor vehicle accident who suffered bilateral renal injuries. Note the wedge-shaped area of non-enhancement (*arrow*) along the anterolateral border of the right kidney.

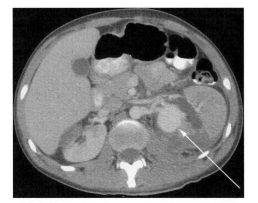

Fig. 7. Grade 4 renal injury: pseudoaneurysm. Contrast-enhanced CT of patient involved in a high-speed motor vehicle accident. Patient suffered substantial drop in hematocrit 20 days after initial injury and repeat CT demonstrated a new well-circumscribed left renal artery pseudoaneurysm (*arrow*).

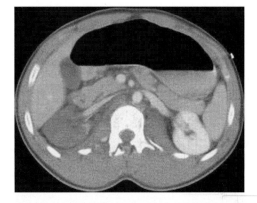

Fig. 9. Grade 5 renal injury: main renal artery thrombosis. Contrast-enhanced CT of a patient involved in a motor vehicle collision demonstrates a non-enhancing right kidney. Note the lack of perinephric fluid. (*From* Smith JK, Kenney PJ. Imaging of renal trauma. Radiologic Clinics of North America 2003;41(5):1019–35.)

has been shown to successfully identify free intraperitoneal fluid and possible organ injury [10], it cannot differentiate between blood, extravasated urine, and other types of free fluid. This is a crucial distinction with regard to genitourinary trauma. Furthermore, as many as 65% of isolated renal injuries will not have associated free fluid [11]. Overall, US has been shown to be less sensitive compared with CT for the identification of renal injuries [12,13]. If ultrasonography suggests a renal injury, or if US is negative and there is significant hematuria, the patient should undergo CT provided the patient is stable.

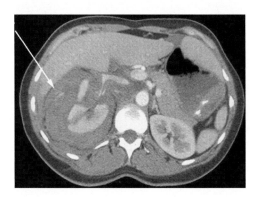

Fig. 8. Grade 5 renal injury: active extravasation. Contrast-enhanced CT scan of a patient involved in a motor vehicle accident with a right renal laceration. Note the waterfall-shaped area of vascular contrast extravasation (*arrow*) within the perinephric hematoma.

Magnetic resonance imaging with gadolinium can provide detailed images with regard to renal injuries, but simply is not practical in the acute trauma patient. Angiography can be an important adjunct to CT in patients with active vascular extravasation. In cases were there is active extravasation from a renal vessel or delayed hemorrhage from a pseudoaneurysm, angiography with transcatheter embolization has been shown to be successful [14,15].

Intraoperative imaging

Hematuria in the unstable patient undergoing emergent laparotomy still requires immediate assessment. In this situation, a "single-shot" excretory urogram is obtained. A single plain film is taken 10 minutes after intravenous injection of 2 cc/kg of iodinated contrast. Morey and colleagues [16] have shown that the findings from a properly obtained intraoperative excretory urogram safely obviated renal exploration in 32% of patients. They observed no complications and no contrast reactions in this study.

Ureteral injuries

Traumatic ureteral injuries are quite rare, representing less than 1% of all genitourinary traumas [17]. This is partly because the proximal ureter is well protected by the psoas muscle and vertebrae, while the distal ureter is protected by the bony pelvis. Given this fact, a patient must suffer a significant traumatic event to injure the ureter. There is concomitant abdominal organ

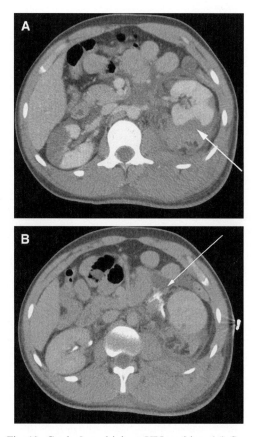

Fig. 10. Grade 5 renal injury: UPJ avulsion. (*A*) Contrast-enhanced CT of a patient involved in a high-speed motor vehicle accident with bilateral renal injuries. Note multiple areas of non-enhancement within the left kidney, which is displaced anteriorly by perinephric fluid (*arrow*). (*B*) Delayed images reveal urinary extravasation from UPJ (*arrow*). No contrast was seen in the distal ureter on lower images.

injury in the vast majority of cases, with small and large bowel injuries seen most frequently [17,18].

Indications for ureteral imaging

About 56% of patients with ureteral injuries are hypotensive on presentation, indicative of the severity of trauma that was incurred rather than the ureteral injury itself [17]. The most recent studies show that hematuria, either gross or microscopic, is present in about 75% to 85% of patients [17,19]. If there is complete ureteral transection or an adynamic segment of ureter, hematuria may not be present. Thus, one must pay particular attention to mechanism of injury

when considering the possibility of a ureteral injury. All stable patients with penetrating injuries require radiographic evaluation. Patients with blunt injuries resulting from rapid deceleration also require radiographic imaging.

Radiographic assessment

Computerized tomography

Contrast-enhanced CT is highly sensitive at detecting urine extravasation, as well as other organ injuries, and should be considered the first mode of imaging for ureteral trauma. As previously stated, it is essential to obtain delayed images about 10 minutes after contrast injection to avoid missing urinary extravasation (see Fig. 11) [6].

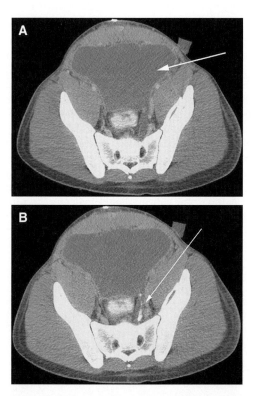

Fig. 11. Distal ureteral injury. This patient suffered a gunshot wound to the abdomen. He underwent exploratory laparotomy and bowel resection, but the distal ureter was not explored. He developed abdominal pain and distention and underwent a contrast-enhanced CT. (*A*) Initial arterial phase demonstrates a large fluid collection in inferior recesses of the peritoneum (*arrow*). (*B*) Delayed image shows extravasation of contrast from distal ureter (*arrow*) into the fluid collection.

Excretory urography

Many patients in whom ureteral injury may be a concern will progress to immediate laparotomy because of instability from other intra-abdominal injuries. In this situation, a "one-shot" excretory urogram may be obtained intraoperatively to assess for possible upper urinary tract injuries. A single film should be taken 10 minutes after intravenous injection of contrast material (see Fig. 12). These studies can sometimes provide sub-optimal visualization of the upper urinary tract. A negative study does not completely remove the possibility of a ureteral injury and surgical exploration should be performed if a ureteral injury is still suspected.

Retrograde pyelography

A retrograde pyelogram has been shown to be extremely sensitive in identifying ureteral injuries [20]. However, it is most often not feasible in the acute trauma setting. We have found it to be a good adjunct to CT-IVP to confirm and further delineate the extent of ureteral injury. It can also be helpful in planning further surgical management of the injury.

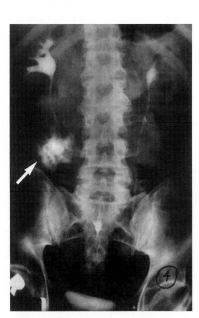

Fig. 12. Excretory urogram of patient who suffered abdominal stab wound. Note there is no contrast distal to the site of extravasation, indicative of complete ureteral transaction. (*From* McAninch JW, Santucci RA. Genitourinary rauma. In: Walsh PC, Retik AB, Vaughan ED, et al, editors. Campbell's urology. 8th edition. Philadelphia: WB Saunders; 2002. p. 3717.)

Bladder injuries

Bladder injury can occur as a result of blunt or penetrating lower abdominal trauma. It is relatively uncommon because of the protection provided by the bony pelvis. However, about 10% of individuals who suffer a pelvic fracture will have a concomitant bladder injury [21]. Proper characterization of these injuries by radiographic imaging is essential to proper management.

Indications for cystography

Almost all patients (95% to 100%) with injury to the bladder will present with gross hematuria [22,23], with the remaining patients having microscopic hematuria [22]. Occasionally there will be no return of urine upon catheterization of the bladder and this situation also demands cystography. Bladder injury is associated with urethral disruption in about 10% to 29% of cases [22]. These patients present with blood at the urethral meatus, the inability to urinate, or perineal ecchymosis. In this situation, a retrograde urethrogram should be performed to evaluate the urethra before catheterization and cystography.

Radiographic assessment

CT cystography

We currently recommend CT cystography as opposed to standard cystography for the evaluation of possible bladder injuries. This approach saves time since almost all patients will undergo CT for evaluation of intra-abdominal organ injury and pelvic fracture. A scan of the lower abdomen and pelvis is obtained after retrograde instillation of 350 cc (or until the patient experiences discomfort) of diluted contrast. A second scan after contrast drainage should also be obtained (see Figs. 13 and 14). It is necessary to dilute the contrast material because undiluted contrast is too dense and will compromise the quality of the obtained images. We have obtained excellent images using 5% dilute solution, but other authors have recommended using even more dilute 2% solution [24]. CT cystogram performed by intravenous injection of contrast, clamping of the Foley catheter, and delayed imaging is not recommended. This technique has been shown to lead to missed injuries [25]. Studies have shown that CT cystography is equally as sensitive as conventional cystography for the detection of bladder injuries [24,26].

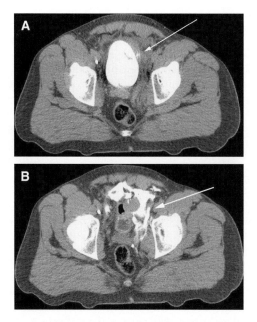

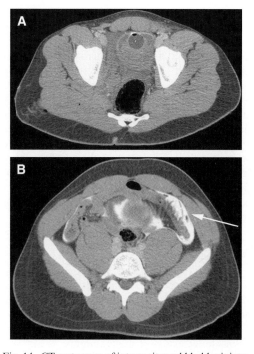

Fig. 13. CT cystogram of extraperitoneal bladder injury. (*A*) Initial CT after filling bladder shows small amount of extravasation (*arrow*) from left lateral wall of bladder. (*B*) Repeat scan after drainage confirms extraperitoneal extravasation (*arrow*).

Fig. 14. CT cystogram of intraperitoneal bladder injury. (*A*) Initial scan through pelvis reveal catheter balloon with bladder. (*B*) Scan after instillation of contrast through catheter reveals intraperitoneal extravasation of contrast. Note that bowel loops are outlined by the extravasated contrast (*arrow*).

Conventional cystography

Conventional retrograde cystography, with plain abdominal x-ray and drainage films, has been shown to have 100% accuracy in diagnosing significant bladder injuries [23]. To perform properly, approximately 350 cc of contrast are instilled in the bladder via a catheter and a plain abdominal film is obtained in the anteroposterior projection. The bladder is then emptied and a second post drainage film is obtained. This second film is essential, as approximately 13% of bladder injuries are detected on the drainage film [23].

An extraperitoneal rupture routinely demonstrates extravasated contrast confined to the pelvis, although it may track into the retroperitoneal space. The extravasated contrast often appears as flame-like wisps or linear streaks (see Fig. 15). With an intraperitoneal rupture, the contrast extravasates throughout the peritoneal cavity. It is typically visible in the paracolic gutters and outlining loops of bowel (see Fig. 16).

Urethral injuries

Traumatic injuries to the urethra occur in approximately 10% of patients who suffer pelvic fractures [27]. They are extremely rare in female

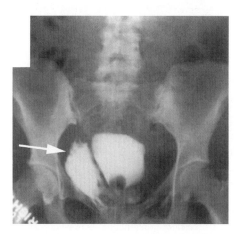

Fig. 15. Cystogram of extraperitoneal bladder injury. Extravasated contrast appears as a flame-like wisp contained within the extraperitoneal space (*arrow*). (*From* McAninch JW, Santucci RA. Genitourinary trauma. In: Walsh PC, et al, editors. Campbell's urology. 8th edition. Philadelphia: WB Saunders; 2002. p. 3722.)

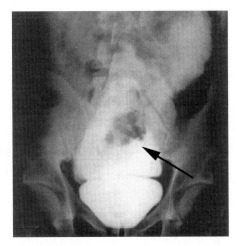

Fig. 16. Cystogram of intraperitoneal bladder injury. Note extravasated contrast within peritoneal cavity, outlining loops of bowel (*dark arrow*). (*From* McAninch JW, Santucci RA. Genitourinary trauma. In: Walsh PC, Retik AB, Vaughan ED, et al, editors. Campbell's urology. 8th edition. Philadelphia: WB Saunders; 2002. p. 3722.)

patients because of the hypermobility of the urethra and lack of bony attachments. This diagnosis should be considered in all patients who present with pelvic fractures.

Indications for imaging

The most common clinical findings in patients with urethral injuries are gross hematuria or blood at the urethral meatus. Occasionally, a patient may present with a full bladder and an inability to urinate. On physical examination, there can be perineal/scrotal swelling and ecchymosis resulting from extravasation of blood. A perineal "butterfly hematoma" is classically described. Digital rectal examination is also important and can reveal an absent or "high-riding" prostate. If any of the above findings are noted on presentation, a retrograde urethrogram (RUG) is indicated. These classic findings may not be present initially and the possibility of a urethral injury is appreciated only after the trauma team is unable to place a urethral catheter. Again, the diagnosis should then be confirmed with a RUG.

Retrograde urethrogram

The ideal positioning for performing a retrograde urethrogram is with the patient in the oblique position with the penis stretched perpendicular to the femur. Multiple techniques have been described in the literature [28]. Some urologists prefer to perform the instillation of contrast using a catheter-tip bulb syringe or a Brodney clamp (Fig. 17). Alternatively, a 14-Fr Foley catheter can be inserted at the meatus and the balloon then inflated in the fossa navicularis with 2 to 3 cc of sterile water. A Toomey syringe is then used to administer 30 to 40 cc of water-soluble contrast and a plain film is obtained while the last 10 cc is instilled. Complete disruption is demonstrated by extravasation without filling of the bladder (see Fig. 18). Partial filling of the bladder with extravasation is indicative of partial disruption (see Fig. 19). If there is no extravasation, the catheter should be advanced into the bladder and a cystogram should be performed to ensure there is no bladder injury. Of note, concomitant bladder injuries occur in 10% to 29% of patients with a urethral injury [29].

Scrotal trauma

The scrotum and testicles can be subject to both blunt and penetrating injury. The physical examination can vary tremendously from a small area of ecchymosis to massive swelling and discoloration as a result of extensive hemorrhage. We recommend scrotal exploration in all cases where there is a large hematocele or rupture of the tunica albuginea. Scrotal ultrasound can be used as an adjunct to the physical examination. This may reveal a heterogeneous appearance of the testicular parenchyma, suggestive of intratesticular hemorrhage, or disruption of the tunica (see Fig. 20). If the ultrasound is inconclusive, one should still proceed with exploration if the physical examination is grossly abnormal.

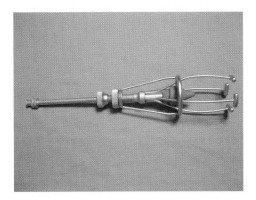

Fig. 17. Modified Brodney clamp.

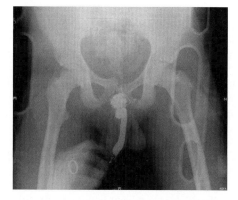

Fig. 18. Retrograde urethrogram of complete urethral disruption. Note that no contrast is seen within the bladder. A catheter was able to be placed with retrograde cystoscopy. Cystogram revealed no evidence of bladder injury.

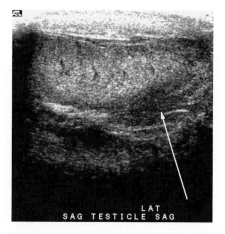

Fig. 20. Scrotal ultrasound of testicular injury. This patient suffered a gunshot wound to the right hemiscrotum. On exam, he had mild tenderness of the right testicle and a small hematoma. Ultrasound shows disruption of the inferior border of the tunica with a heterogeneous appearance of the testicular parenchyma in this region (*arrow*). Exploration revealed a tunical injury and patient underwent partial orchiectomy.

External genital injuries

Penetrating injury to the penis can occur from gunshot or stab wounds, or as a result of self-mutilation. Retrograde urethrography is recommended in all patients, as studies have shown urethral injury in up to 50% of patients [30,31].

Penile "fracture"—corpus cavernosal rupture from blunt trauma to the erect penis—is relatively uncommon. In the United States, the most common cause is striking of the penis on the perineum

or symphysis during intercourse [32]. The patient often reports hearing a "pop." On physical exam, there is almost always penile swelling and ecchymosis and a corporal defect can occasionally be palpated. Some have reported the use of ultrasound to aid in the diagnosis (see Fig. 21) [33], but history and physical exam are in general sufficient to make the diagnosis. Others have reported using cavernosography with excellent sensitivity [34]. This is performed by percutaneously placing a 25-gauge butterfly needle into the corpus cavernosum and injecting contrast material. Fluoroscopy or plain radiography is then used to obtain images. An associated urethral injury is seen in about a third of patients with penile fractures [32]. A retrograde urethrogram should be obtained in all penile fracture patients who present with gross hematuria, blood at the meatus, or with the inability to void.

Summary

All practicing urologists will encounter a wide variety of traumatic injuries in their career, as 3% to 10% of trauma patients have injury to the genitourinary tract [1,2]. In these situations, radiologic imaging is essential for making the correct diagnosis and managing it appropriately. One should choose which radiographic modality

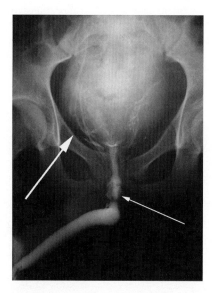

Fig. 19. Retrograde urethrogram of partial urethral disruption (*thin arrow*). Note that there is contrast seen within the bladder (*thick arrow*).

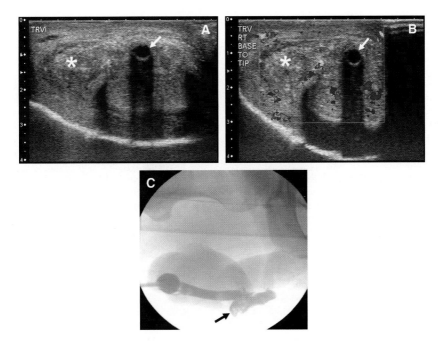

Fig. 21. Ultrasound of penile fracture. This patient presented with loss of penile rigidity, pain, and hematuria after an injury suffered during intercourse. (*A*) Transverse sonogram of the penis shows subcutaneous hematoma of variable echogenicity in continuity with the right corpus cavernosa (asterisk), suggesting a fracture. A Foley catheter (*arrow*) is within the urethra. (*B*) Corresponding color-flow images shows absence of flow within the area of the fracture. (*C*) Retrograde urethrogram shows a rupture of the bulbar urethra. (*From* Bhatt S, Kocakoc E, Rubens DJ, et al. Sonographic evaluation of penile trauma. Journal of Ultrasound Medicine 2005;24:993–1000.)

is appropriate based on the mechanism of injury and patient presentation. All patients with penetrating trauma and hematuria, blunt abdominal trauma with shock or gross hematuria, or a rapid deceleration injury warrant imaging of the urinary tract. Computed tomography is the modality of choice for most situations. Obtaining delayed images is essential in diagnosing the presence of urinary extravasation. Patients with pelvic injuries and gross hematuria should undergo either CT cystography or conventional cystography. Those with blood at the urethral meatus, inability to urinate, perineal/scrotal ecchymosis, or abnormal digital rectal exam should undergo retrograde urethrography. Ultrasound is warranted in patients with scrotal trauma when physical exam is inconclusive. Patients with penetrating trauma to the external genitalia should undergo retrograde urethrography, as should those who suffer blunt trauma to the penis and present with gross hematuria, blood at the meatus, or the inability to void. Using these criteria for imaging should lead to the proper diagnosis and minimize patient morbidity.

Acknowledgments

We acknowledge Michelle E. Goodall, Radiology Applications Specialist, Department of Radiology, MetroHealth Medical Center, for her assistance in gathering the images seen in this text.

References

[1] Carroll PR, McAninch JW. Staging of renal trauma. Urol Clin North Am 1989;16:193–201.

[2] Krieger JN, Algood CB, Mason JT, et al. Urological trauma in the Pacific Northwest: etiology, distribution, management and outcome. J Urol 1984;132:70–3.

[3] Mee SL, McAninch JW, Robinson AL, et al. Radiographic assessment of renal trauma: a 10-year prospective study of patient selection. J Urol 1989;141:1095–8.

[4] Nicolaisen GS, McAninch JW, Marshall GA, et al. Renal trauma: re-evaluation of the indications for radiographic assessment. J Urol 1985;133:183–7.

[5] Miller KS, McAninch JW. Radiographic assessment of renal trauma: our 15-year experience. J Urol 1995;154:352–5.

[6] Brown SL, Elder JS, Spirnak JP. Are pediatric patients more susceptible to major renal injury

from blunt trauma? A comparative study. J Urol 1998;160:138–40.

[7] Perez-Brayfield MR, Gatti JM, Smith EA, et al. Blunt traumatic hematuria in children. Is a simplified algorithm justified? J Urol 2002;167:2543–6.

[8] Brown SL, Hoffman DM, Spirnak JP. Limitations of routine spiral computerized tomography in the evaluation of blunt renal trauma. J Urol 1998;160: 1979–81.

[9] Moore EE, Shackford SR, Pachter HL, et al. Organ injury scaling: spleen, liver, and kidney. J Trauma 1989;29:1664–6.

[10] McKenney KL, Nunez DB Jr, McKenney MG, et al. Sonography as the primary screening technique for blunt abdominal trauma: experience with 899 patients. AJR Am J Roentgenol 1998;170:979–85.

[11] McGahan JP, Richards JR, Jones CD, et al. Use of ultrasonography in the patient with acute renal trauma. J Ultrasound Med 1999;18:207–13.

[12] McGahan JP, Rose J, Coates TL, et al. Use of ultrasonography in the patient with acute abdominal trauma. J Ultrasound Med 1997;16:653–62.

[13] Perry MJ, Porte ME, Urwin GH. Limitations of ultrasound evaluation in acute closed renal trauma. J R Coll Surg Edinb 1997;42:420–2.

[14] Sofocleous CT, Hinrichs C, Hubbi B, et al. Angiographic findings and embolotherapy in renal arterial trauma. Cardiovasc Intervent Radiol 2005;28:39–47.

[15] Giannopoulos A, Manousakas T, Alexopoulou E, et al. Delayed life-threatening haematuria from a renal pseudoaneurysm caused by blunt renal trauma treated with selective embolization. Urol Int 2004;72:352–4.

[16] Morey AF, McAninch JW, Tiller BK, et al. Single shot intraoperative excretory urography for the immediate evaluation of renal trauma. J Urol 1999; 161:1088–92.

[17] Elliott SP, McAninch JW. Ureteral injuries from external violence: the 25-year experience at San Francisco General Hospital. J Urol 2003;170:1213–6.

[18] Medina D, Lavery R, Ross SE, et al. Ureteral trauma: preoperative studies neither predict injury nor prevent missed injuries. J Am Coll Surg 1998; 186:641–4.

[19] Perez-Brayfield MR, Keane TE, Krishnan A, et al. Gunshot wounds to the ureter: a 40-year experience

at Grady Memorial Hospital. J Urol 2001;166: 119–21.

[20] Campbell EW Jr, Filderman PS, Jacobs SC. Ureteral injury due to blunt and penetrating trauma. Urology 1992;40:216–20.

[21] Hochberg E, Stone NN. Bladder rupture associated with pelvic fracture due to blunt trauma. Urology 1993;41:531–3.

[22] Cass AS. The multiple injured patient with bladder trauma. J Trauma 1984;24:731–4.

[23] Carroll PR, McAninch JW. Major bladder trauma: mechanisms of injury and a unified method of diagnosis and repair. J Urol 1984;132:254–7.

[24] Peng MY, Parisky YR, Cornwell EE 3rd, et al. CT cystography versus conventional cystography in evaluation of bladder injury. AJR Am J Roentgenol 1999;173:1269–72.

[25] Haas CA, Brown SL, Spirnak JP. Limitations of routine spiral computerized tomography in the evaluation of bladder trauma. J Urol 1999;162: 51–2.

[26] Deck AJ, Shaves S, Talner L, et al. Current experience with computed tomographic cystography and blunt trauma. World J Surg 2001;25:1592–6.

[27] Glass RE, Flynn JT, King JB, et al. Urethral injury and fractured pelvis. Br J Urol 1978;50:578–82.

[28] Gallentine ML, Morey AF. Imaging of the male urethra for stricture disease. Urol Clin North Am 2002; 29:361–72.

[29] Cass AS, Gleich P, Smith C. Simultaneous bladder and prostatomembranous urethral rupture from external trauma. J Urol 1984;132:907–8.

[30] Miles BJ, Poffenberger RJ, Farah RN, et al. Management of penile gunshot wounds. Urology 1990; 36:318–21.

[31] Cline KJ, Mata JA, Venable DD, et al. Penetrating trauma to the male external genitalia. J Trauma 1998;44:492–4.

[32] Fergany AF, Angermeier KW, Montague DK. Review of Cleveland Clinic experience with penile fracture. Urology 1999;54:352–5.

[33] Koga S, Saito Y, Arakaki Y, et al. Sonography in fracture of the penis. Br J Urol 1993;72:228–9.

[34] Karadeniz T, Topsakal M, Ariman A, et al. Penile fracture: differential diagnosis, management and outcome. Br J Urol 1996;77:279–81.

ELSEVIER
SAUNDERS

Urol Clin N Am 33 (2006) 377–396

UROLOGIC
CLINICS
of North America

The Role of Imaging in the Surveillance of Urologic Malignancies

Timothy J. Bradford, MD, James E. Montie, MD, Khaled S. Hafez, MD*

Department of Urology, University of Michigan Medical Center, 1500 East Medical Center Drive, Ann Arbor, MI 48109-0330, USA

Urologic malignancies are common, accounting for approximately 25% of all new cancer cases in the United States [1]. In addition, urologic malignancies often have prolonged latent periods and high survival rates following treatment. Because of these factors, many patients with urologic malignancies require long-term surveillance to detect progression or recurrence as early as possible and provide adjuvant or salvage therapy. The urologist is faced with the task of balancing patient safety and cost-effectiveness, while finding the most practical follow-up regimen. In addition to regular physical examinations and laboratory studies, imaging modalities such as ultrasonography, plain film radiography, CT, and MRI are essential to cancer surveillance strategies. For each urologic malignancy, this article reviews the commonly used radiologic techniques for surveillance and offers recommended follow-up schedules.

Prostate cancer

Prostate cancer remains the most common malignancy to affect males in the United States, with an estimated 232,090 new cases in 2005, accounting for 33% of new male cancer cases [1]. For all stages, the 10- and 15-year survival rates have been reported to be 92% and 61%, respectively [1]. Recent studies also have shown that the percentage of men diagnosed with low-risk prostate cancer has increased from 29.8% from 1989 to 1992 to 45.3% from 1999 to 2001 [2].

These factors combined suggest that most men diagnosed with prostate cancer will require many years of follow-up. Although the role of imaging in the surveillance of prostate cancer is not clearly defined, studies including transrectal ultrasounds, bone scans and CT scans, as well as newer imaging modalities such as positron emission tomography (PET) and radioimmunoscintigraphy are used commonly. In most cases, however, the presence or absence of other signs and symptoms of cancer recurrence, such as biochemical failure or bone pain, determine in large part the usefulness of radiologic studies.

Watchful waiting

Along with prostate-specific antigen (PSA) monitoring, the purpose of radiologic surveillance during watchful waiting is to detect disease progression that may benefit from intervention as early as possible to provide the patient with options for palliative or potentially curative treatment. The most common imaging techniques routinely used in watchful waiting protocols are transrectal ultrasonography (TRUS) and bone scans. Although there are no definitive guidelines regarding the use of either of these studies during watchful waiting, a review of the literature reveals several common practice patterns. Several watchful waiting studies have included TRUS examinations every 6 to 12 months [3–5], and some have recommended that annual TRUS examinations be included in the standard watchful waiting protocol [6]. Hruby and colleagues, however, found little value for serial TRUS in watchful waiting, with no correlation seen between PSA change and TRUS examinations in the 136 men they

* Corresponding author.
E-mail address: khafez@med.umich.edu (K.S. Hafez).

studied [7]. The more common use of TRUS among watchful waiting protocols has been to facilitate repeat biopsies, which typically are performed 12 to 18 months after diagnosis and often yearly thereafter [3–6,8–10]. There is, however, no standard and no strong evidence as to the benefit of serial TRUS examinations or repeat biopsies.

Similarly, bone scans are performed at different intervals and for slightly different indications among the watchful waiting protocols. Although several watchful waiting studies obtained bone scans on an annual or semiannual basis [4,5,11], current recommendations generally agree that bone scans should be performed only when clinically indicated by symptoms of bone pain or elevated PSA values [6,8]. There is some disagreement, however, as to what PSA level warrants the acquisition of a bone scan. It has been reported that for PSA values of 20 to 50 ng/mL, the rate of positive bone scans is approximately 8%, while the rate is 16% for PSA values greater than 50 ng/mL [12]. In addition, PSA values greater than 50 ng/mL have been shown to often be associated with radiologic evidence of skeletal metastasis [13]. After evaluating a series of 244 men with clinical stage T1-2b prostate cancer on a watchful waiting protocol, Yap and colleagues recommended that bone scans should be obtained only when PSA values exceed 15 ng/mL because of the low yield below this level [14]. There are also no standard recommendations regarding a rising PSA, although a significant increase in PSA likely should be evaluated with a bone scan.

Hormonal therapy

Radiologic surveillance of those men on hormonal therapy for prostate cancer consists mainly of periodic bone scans. It has been suggested that routine imaging is not needed in low-risk patients who have stable PSA values and no clinical evidence of disease progression [8,15]. Rising PSA values or clinical symptoms, however, are indications to obtain a bone scan and consider a CT scan [8]. In addition, for patients who have high-risk T3-4 disease, Messing and Thompson suggest bone scans be performed every 12 months for those with a Gleason score of less than or equal to 7 and PSA values less than 15 ng/mL, and every 6 months for those with Gleason score 8 to 10 or PSA values greater than 15 ng/mL [8]. For those with metastatic disease receiving hormonal therapy, bone scans are recommended every 6 months

for those with a PSA nadir less than 2.0 ng/mL, and every 3 months for those with PSA nadir greater than 2.0 ng/mL [8]. In addition, those men receiving hormonal therapy should be considered for baseline and periodic bone mineral density studies if prolonged treatment is anticipated [8].

Radical prostatectomy

The purpose of radiologic imaging following radical prostatectomy (RP) is early detection of local or distant recurrences to initiate salvage radiotherapy or androgen deprivation if appropriate. Among those with recurrence after RP, Pound and colleagues reported that 45% of patients experienced the recurrence within the first 2 years, 77% within the first 5 years, and 23% after 6 years [16]. Imaging modalities, such as bone scans, CT scans, PET, and radioimmunoscintigraphy have been used to detect and localize recurrent disease with varying degrees of success, but none have proven to be as valuable as following post-RP PSA levels. Reporting on a series of 1916 men following RP, Pound and colleagues found no recurrences in the absence of a detectable PSA, and therefore suggested that imaging is unnecessary in postprostatectomy patients with an undetectable PSA and no other clinical evidence of recurrence [17]. In the setting of increasing PSA levels following RP, however, imaging studies often are needed to localize the site of recurrence. The National Comprehensive Cancer Network (NCCN) defines biochemical recurrence after RP as PSA greater than 0.3 ng/mL and rising on two or more determinations. [10]

As in watchful waiting protocols, the role of TRUS following RP to detect local recurrence lies mainly in the facilitation of site-directed biopsies of the prostatic fossa. Several studies were reviewed by Nelson and Lepor, who found that the average positive biopsy rate was 57% [18]. Even if this information was used to guide recommendations for local salvage radiotherapy, multiple studies have shown similar results for salvage treatment whether done empirically, in the setting of a negative biopsy, or in response to a positive biopsy [19–22]. Therefore, TRUS-guided prostatic fossa biopsy is not recommended in the routine evaluation of biochemical failure following RP [18].

Currently, the most commonly used imaging modality for surveillance following RP is that of radionuclide bone scintigraphy, or bone scans.

Although routine bone scans are not recommended as part of surveillance in the absence of biochemical failure, several authors have suggested that a baseline bone scan may be useful [23,24]. The one indication for a bone scan that generally is agreed upon is the development of bone pain or other symptoms suggestive of skeletal metastases [10,23–25]. In the absence of clinical symptoms, however, the value of this test depends significantly on the PSA levels at which it is performed. Cher and colleagues reported on the probability of a positive bone scan after RP and concluded that bone scintigraphy has little utility until PSA values rise above 30 to 40 ng/mL [26]. After reviewing 12 studies on bone scintigraphy and PSA levels, Nelson and Lepor recommended that bone scans are not necessary for asymptomatic patients with a PSA less than 10 ng/mL [18]. The 2005 NCCN guidelines suggest a bone scan for postprostatectomy patients who have PSA values greater than 0.3 ng/mL and rising on two or more determinations [10]. The European Association of Urology (EAU) recommends that bone scans may be delayed until PSA levels exceed 20 ng/mL [15]. Finally, in a recent American Urological Association (AUA) Update, Theodorescu and colleagues recommended yearly bone scans for PSA levels greater than 20 ng/mL [24].

The role of CT scans for surveillance following RP is not defined well, but they may have utility in patients who have increasing PSA values and no documented site of recurrence [27]. Kramer and colleagues found that CT scans were positive in only 36% of 22 biopsy-confirmed local recurrences; therefore, they did not recommend that CT scanning be included in routine follow-up after RP [28]. Seltzer and colleagues, however, suggested some utility of CT scans following RP in those patients with PSA values greater than 4 ng/mL or PSA velocity greater than 0.2 ng/mL/month [29]. The EAU also suggests delaying CT scans in asymptomatic patients until PSA values exceed 4 ng/mL [15]. There has been little reported on the value of MRI for detection of recurrent disease. In a prospective analysis of 41 postprostatectomy patients who underwent MRI with a transrectal surface coil, however, Silverman and Krebs reported 100% sensitivity and 100% specificity for the detection of local recurrence [30]. Several studies also have demonstrated limited value of MRI in the detection of bone metastases [31,32].

PET scanning is another imaging modality that has been used with some success for surveillance following RP. The major potential role for PET scanning is distinguishing postoperative fibrosis from residual or recurrent disease after RP, which CT is unable to accomplish [33]. Although several studies have shown some utility for 18F-fluorodeoxyglucose (FDG) PET scanning in this setting [34,35], Hofer and colleagues found that FDG-PET was unable to distinguish fibrosis from local recurrence following RP [36]. Using the ^{11}C-acetate isotope however, Kotzerke and colleagues reported positive PET scans in 15 of 18 patients with biopsy-proven local recurrence, and negative scans in 13 of 13 biopsy-negative patients [37]. Another potential application for PET scanning could be to localize and quantify response to treatment [38].

Radioimmunoscintigraphy with the ProstaScint scan (Cytogen Corp., Princeton, NJ) uses a radiolabeled antibody directed against prostate-specific membrane antigen (PSMA) to detect residual local or recurrent disease. Elgamal and colleagues compared eight studies, including their own, and reported sensitivities of 44% to 92% and specificities of 36% to 86% [39]. Likewise, Nelson and Lepor found wide variations in positive predictive values among nine more recent studies [18]. The most clinically useful role for ProstaScint scanning may be to exclude those with extensive systemic disease on imaging from local salvage radiotherapy [18]. Most recommend the use of ProstaScint scans only in the setting of a persistently elevated or rising PSA level with no source identifiable by other imaging modalities or TRUS-guided biopsy [27].

External beam radiotherapy

As is the case following RP, the value of imaging studies performed following external beam radiotherapy (EBRT) depends largely on the PSA value, which is the most common sign of recurrence [40]. The definition of biochemical failure most widely used following EBRT is three consecutive increases in PSA, which was proposed by the American Society for Therapeutic Radiology and Oncology (ASTRO) in 1997 [41]. Transrectal ultrasound imaging has been used to a limited extent to detect local recurrences following EBRT; however, sensitivity of TRUS alone to detect persistent malignancy following EBRT has been reported to be approximately 50% [27]. Again, TRUS is most useful in guiding biopsies in the setting of PSA failure following EBRT. The NCCN guidelines recommend biopsy only for those with PSA failure who are candidates for local therapy [10]. Likewise, the consensus recommendation by ASTRO in 1997 was that post-EBRT prostate biopsies not be performed unless salvage procedures were being considered [42].

In general, bone scans are used following EBRT in much the same way as following RP. In the setting of PSA failure, bone scans are recommended to distinguish residual local disease from metastasis [10,40]. Studies of men who have newly diagnosed prostate cancer, however, have shown that fewer than 10% of bone scans are positive in those men with PSA values less than 20 ng/mL and Gleason scores greater than 7, or in those with PSA values less than 50 ng/mL and Gleason scores less than 8 [43]. Therefore, Catton and colleagues have suggested that bone scans are of little value in patients who have very low PSA levels [40]. Although there are no specific guidelines for the use of CT or MRI following EBRT, the NCCN and EUA guidelines suggest that these tests may be useful in evaluating PSA failure [10,15]. The experience with PET and ProstaScint scanning following EBRT is limited. In a large multi-center retrospective study of 340 patients who underwent ProstaScint scans following EBRT, Sodee and colleagues found an association between PSA levels and the detection of ProstaScint activity in the prostate bed [44]. The current role of ProstaScint scanning following EBRT, however, is not well-defined.

Brachytherapy

Following brachytherapy (BT), the American Brachytherapy Society (ABS) recommends that adequate dose and coverage of the prostate be evaluated with postimplant dosimetry [45,46]. Post-implant dosimetry may be obtained using plain films, CT or MRI, but CT is the recommended and most commonly used modality [46,47]. The time interval at which dosimetry should be performed following brachytherapy is controversial, ranging from 24 hours to 4 weeks [46]. For this reason, the ABS recommends that each institution perform postimplant dosimetry at a consistent postoperative interval, which should be specified in the dosimetry report [46].

Evaluation of the postvoid residual by ultrasonography has been recommended 6 to 8 weeks following BT [24,47]. Although the role of routine prostate biopsies following BT is unclear in the absence of PSA failure, Theodorescu and colleagues recommend the same guidelines be followed as described for post-EBRT biopsies [24]. Likewise,

bone scans are recommended only in the setting of clinical symptoms or PSA failure [24].

Cryotherapy

Routine imaging is not required following cryotherapy in the absence of rising PSA values [48]. Transrectal ultrasonography and prostate biopsies, however, often are performed during routine surveillance [48]. After cryotherapy, the treated prostate appears fuzzy on ultrasound secondary to cell death, so TRUS can therefore be used to monitor areas not adequately frozen during initial treatment and hypoechoic lesions suspicious for recurrence [27]. In the event of PSA failure, the various imaging modalities previously described can be used.

Renal cell carcinoma

During 2005, an estimated 36,160 new cases of kidney cancer were diagnosed in the United States, and an estimated 13,180 people died of the disease [1]. Among those treated for localized disease, 25% to 50% may develop metastatic disease [49–51]. Furthermore, numerous studies have suggested that recurrent or metastatic disease is most likely to occur within 2 to 3 years of initial therapy [52–58]. Given the potential survival benefit of surgical resection of metastases with or without immunotherapy in selected patients [59–63], close surveillance and early detection of metastatic disease are critical.

Watchful waiting and minimally invasive therapy

Widespread use of diagnostic imaging such as ultrasonography and CT scans has led to an increase in the detection of incidental renal masses [64]. For many patients who have multiple medical comorbidities, watchful waiting has been offered as an alternative to surgical excision. The imaging modality most commonly used for surveillance is CT, although ultrasounds and MR scans also are employed frequently. Although there is no consensus recommendation on the frequency of imaging, intervals of 6 months to 1 year are used most commonly [65–67].

In addition to surveillance, patients may be offered minimally invasive procedures such as cryosurgery or radio frequency ablation (RFA) for selected tumors as an alternative to surgery. After renal cryoablation, patients have been followed with serial MR scans performed within several days of the surgery, then at 3, 6, and 12 months, and yearly thereafter [68,69]. The ablated lesions typically decrease in size over time. In their series, Gill and colleagues routinely obtained a CT-guided biopsy of the lesion 6 months after treatment and considered the lack of enhancement of the cryoablated tumor as the measure of successful cryoablation [68]. After RFA, Matsumoto and colleagues reported that successfully treated tumors were characterized by lack of contrast enhancement, shrinkage, and variable fat infiltration surrounding the ablated tumor [70]. In their series, CT scans were performed at 6 weeks, 3 months, 6 months, and every 6 months thereafter following the procedure. In a recent report, McDougal and colleagues performed CT scans within 1 month following RFA, then at 3 months, 6 months, and at 6- to 12-month intervals thereafter [71]. Treatment failure was defined as any lesion that enhanced more than 10 to 15 Hounsfield units after contrast administration. In both studies, MR scans were used for patients who had renal insufficiency or contrast allergy.

Radical nephrectomy

Recent guidelines for radiologic surveillance after radical and partial nephrectomy have focused on prognostic factors and their impact on disease recurrence to tailor an individualized follow-up strategy for every patient. In a study of 1864 patients who underwent partial or radical nephrectomy, Frank and colleagues suggested that commonly used prognostic factors, such as stage and grade, were of variable utility in predicting metastasis to different sites and suggested that this information should be used to guide follow-up [72]. Given that the most common sites of metastasis are lung, bone, and the abdomen, the imaging studies used following treatment for renal cell carcinoma focus on these areas.

Considerable variability exists among the studies regarding the percentage of lung recurrences detectable by symptoms alone, ranging from 6.7% to 74% [53,55–57]. The use of chest radiographs to detect lung metastasis is therefore common among most surveillance protocols, although some recommend the use of chest CT because of its ability to detect smaller nodules [52]. Sandock and colleagues reported that all patients in their series with pulmonary metastases had lesions identifiable by plain chest radiograph [57]. The main area of disagreement with regards to the use of chest radiographs is how often they should be obtained in patients after treatment for T1

disease. Although some suggest that chest radiographs are not needed in the postoperative surveillance of T1 lesions [56,57,73], most agree that a chest radiograph should be obtained every 6 to 12 months [25,55,58,74,75]. For stage T2 lesions, most recommend a chest radiograph every 6 months for 2 to 5 years, and then annually thereafter [25,55–57,74,75]. For T3 lesions, several recommend obtaining a chest radiograph at 3 to 4 months postoperatively [25,55,56,75], then every 4 to 6 months for 3 to 5 years, and then annually thereafter [25,55–58,73–75]. Gofrit and colleagues recommend that those with tumors larger than 4 cm should undergo chest CT every 6 months for 5 years and annually thereafter [52]. Others have developed risk groups based on prognostic factors and have made recommendations that high-risk patients be followed with a chest CT every 6 months for 3 years and annually thereafter [54]. Currently, however, most recommend chest CT only for evaluating an abnormal chest radiograph.

The other imaging modality commonly used in routine surveillance following radical nephrectomy is abdominal/pelvic CT. Although only 1.4% to 11% of abdominal metastases are detected by CT alone in the absence of symptoms or abnormal serum studies [55–58], most protocols still include scheduled CT scans of the abdomen and pelvis with and without intravenous contrast based on pathologic stage. Among seven recently suggested protocols, only two recommend baseline CT scans 3 to 6 months postoperatively for all stages [74,75]. While there is agreement that CT scans should be performed to evaluate symptoms or abnormal serum studies, only one protocol calls for routine CT scans in T1 disease [74], and only two studies recommend scheduled CT scans for T2 disease [55,74]. Janzen and colleagues recommend that patients designated as intermediate risk, including some patients who have T1 and T2 disease, undergo CT scans every other year [54]. For those patients who have T3 disease, all but one study [57] recommend scheduled CT scans, with the interval between scans ranging from every 6 months to every other year [54–56,58,74,75]. Whereas one protocol suggests that CT scans do not need to be performed routinely after 1 year [56], others recommend that they be performed indefinitely [54,58,74,75]. The latest recurrence for all stages has been reported to range from 84 months to 144 months [52,55–58]. Therefore, for those patients with T3 or T4 disease and a reasonable life expectancy, surveillance should be lifelong.

Metastases to the bone or brain are very rare in the absence of symptoms or serum abnormalities. Several studies have shown that bone scans are of little value in the preoperative metastatic evaluation of patients with renal cell carcinoma [76,77]. Furthermore, in three series of patients following radical nephrectomy, all patients with bone or brain metastases had either symptoms or abnormal serum studies [55–57]. Therefore, bone scans and head CTs are recommended only in the evaluation of symptoms or serum studies suggestive of metastasis.

PET scans also have been implemented in the surveillance of postnephrectomy patients with considerable success. In fact, the use of PET scans has been reported to affect patient management in up to 40% of cases [78]. Hoh and colleagues demonstrated superior efficacy of PET scans over CT scans in monitoring the response to interleukin 2-based therapy [79]. Ramdave and colleagues reported an accuracy of 100% when using PET to detect local recurrence or metastasis in a small series [80]. In particular, PET was superior to CT in differentiating local recurrence from fibrosis or necrosis. PET offers an additional advantage over CT in that it is a whole body scan, and therefore it may detect metastases that otherwise would have been missed. Although the role of PET in the surveillance of renal cell carcinoma is still evolving, there is potential for future use.

Partial nephrectomy

Nephron-sparing surgery has become much more common in urologic practice over the last decade. Local recurrence rates following partial

nephrectomy have been reported to range from 2% to 10% [81]. Reporting on a series of 327 patients who underwent nephron-sparing surgery, Hafez and colleagues suggested that patients undergoing partial nephrectomy for T1 disease require no postoperative imaging [53]. In contrast, they recommended that patients who had T2 disease undergo yearly chest radiograph and CT of the abdomen and pelvis with and without contrast every 2 years, while those who have T3 disease undergo CT every 6 months for the first 2 years and every 2 years thereafter. Since the study by Hafez and colleagues, however, the TNM system has been modified to change the definition of T1 tumors from less than 2.5 cm to less than 7 cm. Therefore, Evans has suggested that tumors smaller than 2.5 cm need no postoperative imaging, while the remainder of T1 and T2 lesions should be followed postoperatively with an annual chest radiograph and CT scan every 2 years [25]. For those who have T3 disease, abdominal/pelvic CT and chest radiograph are recommended every 6 months for 2 years and every 2 years thereafter. As is the case following radical nephrectomy, bone scans and head CTs are recommended following partial nephrectomy only in the evaluation of symptoms or abnormal serum studies.

Recommended radiologic surveillance following radical or partial nephrectomy for renal cell carcinoma is shown in Table 1.

Testicular cancer

Although testicular cancer is a relatively rare neoplasm, accounting for approximately 1% of all male cancers, it is the most commonly diagnosed

Table 1
Recommended radiologic surveillance following radical/partial nephrectomy for renal cell carcinoma

Disease stage	Year 1	Year 2–5	Year 5–10	> 10 Years
Stage T1				
Chest radiograph	Once yearly	Once yearly	Once yearly	None
Abdominal/pelvic CT/MRI	Baseline 3 mo postoperatively	Once every 2 years	None	None
Stage T2				
Chest radiograph	Once yearly	Once yearly	Once yearly	None
Abdominal/pelvic CT/MRI	Baseline 3 mo postoperatively	Once yearly	Once every 2 years	None
Stage T3–4				
Chest radiograph	Once yearly	Once yearly	Once yearly	Once yearly
Abdominal/pelvic CT/MRI	Once every 3 months	Every 6 months for years 2–3 then once yearly	Once yearly	Once every 2 years

Abdominal/pelvic CT scan with and without intravenous contrast or MRI.

malignancy in developed countries among men aged 15 to 44 years [82,83]. Testicular germ cell tumors (GCTs) generally are characterized as either seminoma, which in its pure form accounts for approximately 35% to 70% of all testicular GCTs, or nonseminoma germ cell tumors (NSGCTs) [84].

Seminoma

Although stage 1 seminoma classically has been treated with radical orchiectomy followed by adjuvant retroperitoneal radiotherapy, active surveillance in lieu of radiotherapy has become an increasingly popular option over the last 20 years. This can be contributed in part to the concern over an increased risk for second malignancies following radiotherapy [85–88] and the high success rates for salvage treatment of recurrence. Several series have evaluated the efficacy of surveillance following orchiectomy and reported relapse rates ranging from 13% to 19% at a median of 13 to 17 months [89–94]. Overall, however, surveillance following orchiectomy for stage 1 seminoma appears to be a reasonable option in well-motivated, low-risk, compliant patients who wish to avoid the potential morbidity of retroperitoneal radiotherapy.

Surveillance focuses on detecting subclinical disease in the chest and abdomen, and is initially very frequent given that most recurrences occur in the first several years. The NCCN guidelines recommend abdominal/pelvic CT every 3 to 4 months for 3 years, then every 6 months for years 4 through 7, then annually thereafter up to 10 years, with chest radiograph performed at alternate visits [95]. Others recommend more intensive surveillance initially, including chest radiograph every 1 to 2 months in the first year [25,74,96,97]. Most agree that CT of the abdomen and pelvis should be performed every 3 to 4 months for the first 3 years and every 6 months for several years thereafter [74,95,96]. Although some centers choose to perform chest CTs instead of chest radiographs, the value of chest CT over chest radiograph has been questioned [98], and most protocols recommend chest radiograph.

Because of the lower recurrence rate (3% to 6%), especially in the abdomen, the follow-up of stage 1 seminoma treated with radiotherapy after orchiectomy is less intensive than for those on surveillance [99–101]. The NCCN guidelines recommend chest radiographs every 3 to 4 months for 1 year, then every 6 months for 1 year, then

annually thereafter [95]. A pelvic CT is recommended every year for 3 years for those who have undergone para-aortic radiotherapy only. Others recommend chest radiographs every 2 to 6 months for the first year and every 3 to 6 months for years 2 through 5 [25,74,96,97]. Although several protocols recommend annual abdominal or abdominal/pelvic CT scans for 3 to 5 years [25,96], others suggest that a baseline abdominal/pelvic CT may be obtained after radiotherapy and only as clinically indicated thereafter [74,97]. Again, length of surveillance has not been established, with recommendations ranging from 5 years [25,96], to 10 years [97], to indefinitely [74,95].

Stage 2A and 2B seminomas are generally categorized together for follow-up purposes. Based on recurrence patterns, the NCCN recommends obtaining a chest radiograph every 3 to 4 months for 3 years, every 6 months for year 4, and annually thereafter [95]. Abdominal/pelvic CT is recommended at 4 months following treatment and only as clinically indicated thereafter. Theodorescu and colleagues recommend the same surveillance for stage 2A/B as for stage 1 following radiotherapy, which includes a baseline CT and chest radiographs every 2 months for the first year, every 3 months for the second year, every 4 months for years 3 and 4, every 6 months for year 5, and annually thereafter [74]. They do, however, suggest that CT scans should be performed every 4 months for 2 years and annually thereafter in those who do not receive hockey stick pattern radiation. The EAU's guidelines are very similar, with frequent chest radiographs for the first 3 to 5 years and a baseline CT after treatment [96].

Advanced disease (stages 2C/3) is present in approximately 25% to 30% of patients with seminoma at the time of presentation [102]. Residual tumor has been found in up to 30% of postchemotherapy masses 3 cm or greater [103]. Given the frequency of residual masses and the possibility of viable tumor, close follow-up is warranted in these patients to monitor for progression. For stage 2C and stage 3 disease, the NCCN guidelines recommend CT of the abdomen and pelvis at month 4 of year 1 [95]. If the CT does not show a residual mass, the NCCN guidelines recommend chest radiograph every 2 months for year 1, every 3 months for year 2, every 4 months for year 3, every 6 months for year 4, and annually thereafter, with abdominal/pelvic CT every 3 months until stable. In the presence of a residual mass, the NCCN recommends obtaining a PET scan. The EAU guidelines and Theodorescu and colleagues recommend more frequent chest radiographs initially but CTs only as indicated or every 6 months, respectively [74,96]. The exception is that when the baseline CT reveals a mass of greater than 3 cm, both recommend that the appropriate CT should be repeated at 2 and 4 months to verify that the mass continues to regress [74,96]. Chest and brain CTs are recommended only when there is an abnormality on chest radiograph, or neurological symptoms, respectively [74,96].

The use of PET scans for surveillance in patients treated for germ cell tumors (in large part because of its ability to distinguish neoplasm from normal tissue based on glucose use) has been evaluated by multiple studies. Several limitations, however, have prevented PET from gaining wide acceptance. Notably, inflammatory and granulomatous tissues can produce false-positive results; lesions less than 1 cm are often not detected, and mature teratoma is not distinguishable from necrotic or normal tissue [104]. Several studies have reported limited utility of PET scans in seminoma patients following chemotherapy, citing false-positive and false-negative results, and no influence on clinical management [105,106]. More recently, however, De Santis and colleagues reported on a prospective multi-center trial of 51 postchemotherapy patients with metastatic seminoma who were evaluated with CT and PET [107]. They reported a specificity, sensitivity, positive predictive value, and negative predictive

value for PET of 100%, 80%, 100%, and 96%, respectively, as compared with 74%, 70%, 37%, and 92%, respectively, for CT. Based on these findings, De Santis and colleagues suggest that PET scans should be part of the standard protocol for surveillance of patients with residual masses following chemotherapy for metastatic seminoma, because those patients with residual lesions greater than 3 cm and negative PET scans may be spared from surgery. Although other studies have not reported such convincing results, many have supported the use of PET as a complementary imaging modality for evaluating residual masses in seminoma patients, mostly because of its superior specificity as compared with CT [108–113]. At this point, it seems that PET may be a useful adjunct to CT in postchemotherapy seminoma patients who have residual masses. Recommended radiologic surveillance for seminoma following orchiectomy with or without radiation or chemotherapy is shown in Tables 2 and 3.

Nonseminoma

Most patients diagnosed with NSGCTs present with clinical stage 1disease [114,115]. For these patients, treatment options include orchiectomy followed by retroperitoneal lymph node dissection (RPLND), chemotherapy, or active surveillance. Recent studies have shown recurrence rates of 24% to 30% among those patients on surveillance [89,97,116–118]. Still, given that approximately 70% of patients who undergo RPLND have negative lymph nodes [118,119], and the high success

Table 2

Recommended radiologic surveillance for seminoma and nonseminomatous germ cell tumors following orchiectomy without radiation, chemotherapy, or retroperitoneal lymph node dissection

Disease Stage	Year 1	Year 2–3	Year 4–7	> 8 years
Clinical stage I seminoma*				
Chest radiograph	Every 3 months	Every 6 months	Once yearly	Every other year to 10 years
Abd/pelvic CT	Every 3 months	Every 4 months	Every 6 months	Once yearly to 10 years
Clinical stage I NSGCT*				
Chest radiograph	Every 2 months	Every 2 months year 2 then every 3 months	Every 4 months year 4, every 6 months year 5 then once yearly	Once yearly
Abd/pelvic CT	Every 2 months	Every 3 months year 2 then every 4 months	Every 6 months year 4 then once yearly	Once yearly

Abdominalpelvic CT scan with and without intravenous contrast.

Abbreviation: NSGCT, nonseminomatous germ cell tumor.

* Serum tumors markers should determine when additional imaging is necessary.

Table 3
Recommended radiologic surveillance for seminoma following orchiectomy and radiation and/or chemotherapy

Disease stage	Year 1	Year 2–3	Year 4–5	> 5 Years
Clinical stage I and IIA/B*				
Chest radiograph	Every 3 months	Every 4 months	Every 6 months	None
Abdominal/pelvic CT	3 mo postoperatively then every 6 months	Every 6 months year 2, then once yearly	Once yearly	None
Clinical stage IIC and III & relapsed stage I and IIA/B*				
Chest radiograph	Every 2 months	Every 2 months year 2, then every 3 months	Every 4 months	Once yearly
Abdominal/pelvic CT	Every 3 months	Every 6 months	Once yearly	None

* Serum tumors markers should determine when additional imaging is necessary.

of salvage chemotherapy, surveillance has become an increasingly popular option for well-motivated and compliant patients. Those patients with risk factors such as the presence of vascular invasion, embryonal carcinoma, or high T stage in the primary tumor specimen, however, may be served better by RPLND. [74]

The use of chest radiographs and chest CTs in the surveillance of stage 1 NSGCT patients has been examined in several series. Harvey and colleagues reported on a series of 168 patients under surveillance for stage 1 NSGCT and concluded that routine surveillance chest CTs were not necessary [98]. Several series also have proposed that routine chest radiographs are unnecessary based on their observations that an abnormal chest radiograph is rarely the only indicator of recurrent disease [120,121]. This is contrary to the results reported by Colls and colleagues, who found that among 248 patients under surveillance, approximately 5% of recurrences were detected by chest radiograph alone [122]. The NCCN guidelines for patients with stage 1 NSGCT on surveillance after radical orchiectomy recommend chest radiograph every 1 to 2 months for the first year, every 2 months for the second year, every 3 months for the third year, every 4 months for the fourth year, every 6 months for the fifth year, and annually thereafter [95]. Abdominal/pelvic CTs are recommended every 2 to 3 months for the first year, every 3 to 4 months for the second year, every 4 months for the third year, every 6 months for the fourth year, and annually thereafter. Several recommendations, including the EAU guidelines, propose that CTs can be spaced out after the second year to once or twice a year [96,97,123,124]. Others suggest that abdominal/pelvic CTs may not be

necessary after year 1 or year 2 unless clinically indicated [116,121]. Although some suggest that follow-up may not be needed beyond 4 years [123], there appear to be enough reported cases of late recurrences to justify surveillance for at least 5 to 10 years, if not for the lifetime of the patient [89,117,125–128].

Several recent series have reported a 10% to 13% relapse rate for patients with pathological stage 1 disease following RPLND [97,118,129]. Most relapses were pulmonary and were detected within the first year. Only one series reported an in-field recurrence, which occurred in one out of 165 patients (0.6%) [129]. Based on these findings, it has been suggested that routine serial abdominal/pelvic CTs are unnecessary in the surveillance of these patients [97]. Most, however, recommend at least a baseline CT at 3 to 6 months after RPLND [74,95,97,130], while others recommend semiannual or annual CTs for at least the first 2 to 5 years [25,96]. Recommendations for obtaining chest radiographs are similar to those for patients on surveillance [74,95–97,130]. Patients who have clinical stage 1 NSGCT who undergo adjuvant chemotherapy instead of RPLND have reported relapse rates of 1% to 5%, and the recurrence is often in the retroperitoneum [130]. Although some suggest that these patients should be followed in the same manner as those patients on surveillance alone [130], several protocols recommend the same schedule as for those patients who undergo RPLND [74,95,96].

Patients who are found to have retroperitoneal disease (stage 2) at the time of RPLND have reported relapse-free survival rates of 97% to 100% when treated with two cycles of adjuvant chemotherapy [118,129,131,132]. In contrast, those who undergo observation only for pathological stage 2 disease after RPLND have reported relapse rates as high as 49% [132]. Because of low recurrence rates, most protocols, including the NCCN guidelines, recommend the same follow-up for those who undergo adjuvant chemotherapy after RPLND for pathological stage 2 as for those with pathological stage 1 disease after RPLND [74,95–97]. This includes frequent chest radiographs, and a baseline CT, with subsequent CTs only as indicated. It also has been suggested that no imaging may be required [130]. On the other hand, those who do not undergo adjuvant chemotherapy require closer surveillance. Some suggest that CT of the suprahilar region and mediastinum should be performed every 4 months for the first 2 years [130]. Others recommend annual CTs if teratoma is found in the retroperitoneum, and semiannual CTs in the first 2 years and annually thereafter if low-volume disease detected at RPLND is managed with observation only [74]. Most agree that chest radiographs should be performed every 1 to 2 months for the first 2 years and less frequently thereafter for these patients [74,96,130]. Patients with clinical stage 2 disease treated with primary chemotherapy after orchiectomy have been reported to have recurrence rates of 11% to 17%, and relapse may occur many years after treatment [133,134]. Routine CTs therefore have been recommended every 4 months during the first 2 years and annually thereafter [130]. Routine chest radiographs have been shown to be of little use in these patients and are therefore unnecessary [133]. The follow-up of patients with stage 3 disease should be comparable to that of patients with stage 2 disease undergoing observation after RPLND.

The role of PET in the surveillance of patients who have NSGCT is defined even more poorly than in patients with seminoma. Although PET scans have been shown to accurately identify viable tumor in postchemotherapy NSGCT patients, it has been unable to differentiate teratoma from necrotic or fibrotic tissue [135]. It has been suggested that PET may be of most use in patients with multiple residual masses, patients with marker-negative disease, and those with conflicting imaging and tumor marker information [104,136]. In these patients, PET eventually may be useful to determine whether surgery is appropriate, but further studies are needed.

In a review of the literature, Herr and colleagues reported that the risk of contralateral metachronous tumor formation in men treated for testis cancer ranges from 1.5% to 3.2% in the United States, and up to 5.2% in Europe [137]. Although significant controversy exists as to whether the contralateral testis should be biopsied [137–139], some have recommended including routine testicular ultrasonography in the follow-up of patients with GCTs [74,140].

Recommended radiologic surveillance for NSGCTs following orchiectomy with or without RPLND or chemotherapy is shown in Tables 2 and 4.

Bladder cancer

Bladder cancer is the second most common urologic malignancy behind prostate cancer, with an estimated 63,210 new cases in the United States in 2005 and 13,180 deaths attributable to this malignancy [1]. At the time of diagnosis, approximately 74% of bladder tumors are superficial; 19% are invasive, and 3% have distant metastasis [1]. Recurrence patterns vary significantly between superficial and invasive bladder cancers, and

Table 4

Recommended radiologic surveillance for nonseminomatous germ cell tumors following orchiectomy and retroperitoneal lymph node dissection and/or chemotherapy

Disease stage	Year 1	Year 2–3	Year 4–5	> 5 Years
Clinical stage I and IIA/B*				
Chest radiograph	Every 2 months	Every 3 months	Every 4 months	Once yearly
Abd/pelvic CT	3 mo postoperatively then every 6 months	Every 6 months	Once yearly	None
Clinical stage IIC and III & relapsed Stage I and IIA/B*				
Chest radiograph	Every month	Every 3 months	Every 4 months	Once yearly
Abd/pelvic CT	Every 3 months	Every 4 months year 2, then 6 months year 3	Once yearly	None

* Serum tumors markers should determine when additional imaging is necessary.

follow-up recommendations therefore are primarily based on pathological stage and grade.

Superficial bladder cancer

There is considerable debate regarding the necessity of upper tract imaging following treatment for superficial bladder cancer in the absence of clinical symptoms or a positive cytology. Some suggest that routine intravenous pyelograms (IVPs) do not improve prognosis, are not cost-effective, and are therefore not justified in the surveillance of patients who have superficial bladder cancer [141–145]. Many recommend IVPs in those who have risk factors for upper tract recurrence, most commonly high-grade disease, multifocality, multiple recurrences, or the presence of carcinoma in situ (CIS) [146–152]. Still others recommend that all patients treated for superficial bladder cancer should be monitored with routine IVPs [25,153–155]. The frequency and duration of surveillance with IVPs ranges from a single baseline study for low-risk patients to annual or semiannual studies for anywhere from 2 years up to the life of the patient [25,146–155]. NCCN guidelines recommend upper tract imaging every 1 to 2 years for the lifetime of the patient in those with high-grade tumors (grade 3), stage T1, or the presence of CIS [156].

Invasive bladder cancer

Following radical cystectomy for bladder cancer, contemporary series report overall recurrence rates ranging from 25% to 46%, with local recurrences occurring in 5% to 19% of patients, distant recurrence occurring in 6% to 22% of patients, and combined local and distant recurrence in 8% to 13% of patients [157–168]. Most recurrences will be detected in the first 2 to 3 years [161,164,169,170]. Relapses most commonly occur in the bone, lung, pelvis, and liver [161,163,169] and have been reported to be symptomatic in 26% to 76% of patients [161,163,171]. The most commonly reported risk factors for recurrence include tumor stage, including lymph node status, grade, and the degree to which pelvic lymphadenectomy is performed [157,158,160,161,163,164, 166,170,172,173]. Metachronous upper tract tumors have been reported to occur in 2.4% to 6.6% of patients at a mean interval of 30 to 80 months after cystectomy [161,163,168,174–179].

As with superficial bladder cancer, several authors suggest that routine upper tract imaging is unnecessary following radical or partial cystectomy, and excretory urography should be performed only in the evaluation of symptoms or a positive cytology [143,145,174,175]. Others have suggested that the combination of renal ultrasound and cytology can replace IVPs for evaluating the upper tracts [24,144,179]. Although some authors recommend excretory urography only for high-risk patients [178,180], most investigators recommend baseline and annual or semiannual upper tract imaging with excretory urography for all patients following cystectomy [25,146,154,156,161,163,169,176,177]. Most recommend that surveillance should be continued for the life of the patient. The options for imaging of the collecting system include IVPs, CT urography, and MR urography. Although IVPs historically have been the standard methodology used, preliminary studies have suggested that CT urography may have higher sensitivity in detecting small upper tract urothelial lesions than excretory urography or even retrograde pyelography [181–185]. Likewise, results for MR urography have been promising [186–189]. The advantage of both CT urography and MR urography over IVPs is that the renal parenchyma, collecting system, abdominal contents, and pelvis can be imaged in one study. In addition to detecting tumor recurrence, these studies are also very effective at demonstrating upper urinary tract complications of urinary diversion, such as calculi or obstruction, 40% to 85% of which may be asymptomatic [161,163]. Furthermore, MR urograms can be used effectively in patients with contrast allergies or poor renal function in whom iodinated contrast material injection may be contraindicated [190]. Disadvantages include the cost and availability of these examinations, and a radiation risk for CT urography that is 1.5 times that of IVPs [191]. Loopography and pouchography also have been used to evaluate the collecting system and urinary diversions following cystectomy. Recently, however, CT urography has been reported to be superior to loopography in its ability to detect urinary calculi, uroepithelial tumors, and extravesicle disease [182].

The need for routine abdominal/pelvic CTs also has been debated in the literature. Some have suggested that CTs are optional in the surveillance of patients following cystectomy [144]. In a review of 382 patients by Slaton and colleagues, only 10% of recurrences were detected by CT scan alone in the absence of symptoms, abnormal serum tests, or disease recurrence at another site [163]. Of those recurrences detected by CT scan,

90% were in patients with pathological T3 disease. Based on these findings, they recommended that abdominal/pelvic CTs be performed only in patients with T3 disease at 6, 12, and 24 months after cystectomy [163]. Following a review of 351 patients, Kuroda and colleagues also suggested that surveillance should be based on stage and recurrence patterns [161]. In their protocol, CT is performed 12 months after cystectomy for patients with T1 disease; at 12, 24, and 36 months for those with T2 disease; and at 4, 8, 12, 18, 24, and 36 months for those with T3 disease or higher. Other recent protocols recommend a baseline study for all postoperative patients, with subsequent CT examinations in patients with nonorgan-confined or high-risk disease every 3 to 6 months for 2 to 4 years, and annually thereafter [24,156]. As previously mentioned, CT urograms offer the advantage of monitoring the collecting system, and the abdominal and pelvic contents, all in one study.

Most protocols agree on the necessity of routine chest radiographs in the follow-up of patients following cystectomy. For stage T1 and T2 disease, most recommend chest radiographs every 6 to 12 months for 2 to 3 years, and annually thereafter [24,25,156,161,163]. For stage T3 disease, chest radiographs are recommended every 3 to 6 months for the first 1 to 5 years, and annually thereafter.

The use of PET scans in bladder cancer has been hampered significantly by the fact that the most commonly used radiotracer (FDG) is highly excreted in the urine and accumulates in the ureters and bladder, making differentiation of lesions in the bladder and adjacent lymph nodes difficult [38]. Although initial studies with FDG PET revealed poor detection of local recurrence, distant metastases still were identified accurately [192,193]. More recently, a new radiotracer, carbon-11 labeled choline, has shown promise because of its minimal urinary tract activity [194]. At this time, however, there is no clear clinical indication for PET scans in the surveillance of patients with bladder cancer. Recommended radiologic surveillance for superficial bladder cancer and invasive bladder cancer following radical cystectomy is shown in Table 5.

Upper tract urothelial carcinoma

Urothelial carcinoma of the upper tracts is a rare disease, accounting for approximately 5% of all urothelial tumors. [195] Among recent series, overall recurrence rates have been reported to range from 8.7% to 42%, with a median time to recurrence of 7 to 18 months [196–203]. Although authors agree that long-term surveillance is required after treatment for upper tract urothelial carcinomas, there is no consensus on which modalities should be used to monitor for recurrence or metastasis. In a study by Chen and colleagues, ureteroscopic cytology with or without biopsy was shown to have a higher sensitivity for detecting recurrence than retrograde pyelography, bladder cytology, or urinalysis [204]. Based on findings such as these, several authors

Table 5
Recommended radiologic surveillance for superficial bladder cancer and following radical cystectomy

Disease stage	Year 1	Year 2–5	Year 5–10	> 10 Years
Stage Ta				
CTU/MRU or IVP	Once yearly	Every 2 years	Every 2 years	None
Stage T1				
CTU/MRU or IVP	Once yearly	Once yearly	Once yearly	None
Organ-confined after radical cystectomy				
Chest radiograph	Once yearly	Once yearly	Once yearly	Once yearly
CTU/MRU	Baseline 3 mo postop	Once yearly	Every 2 years	Abd US every year
Non-organ-confined after cystectomy				
Chest radiograph	Every 3 months	Every 6 months	Once yearly	Once yearly
CTU/MRU	Every 3 months	Every 6 months	Once yearly	Every 2 years & abdominal ultrasound every year

Abbreviations: CTU/MRU, computed tomography urogram or magnetic resonance urogram; IVP, intravenous pyelogram; Abd US, abdominal ultra sound.

recommend routine ureteroscopic evaluation as part of the surveillance program for all patients treated endoscopically for upper tract urothelial carcinoma [200,202,204–206]. On the other hand, many of the recent series reporting on patients managed endoscopically or by nephroureterectomy included only CT urograms, IVPs or ultrasounds in their surveillance programs, with retrograde pyelography or ureteroscopy performed only if indicated by suspicious cytologic or radiographic findings [197–199,207]. Among these series, the frequency of imaging ranged from every 3 to 4 months for the first 2 years and semiannually thereafter, to every 2 years.

Although there are no clear evidence-based guidelines, annual chest radiographs and CT scans of the abdomen have been used by some as part of routine surveillance to detect distant metastases and retroperitoneal recurrence [200,207]. After reviewing the literature, Canfield and colleagues have recommended annual chest radiographs and abdominal CT scans only for patients with high-grade or high-stage disease [195]. For patients treated by nephroureterectomy, the EAU recommends chest radiographs and CTs every 6 months for 2 years and annually thereafter for those with T2 disease or worse, but imaging only for symptoms in those with Ta or T1 disease [205]. Likewise, chest radiographs and CTs are recommended only for evaluating symptoms in those patients treated conservatively by endoscopic resection. NCCN guidelines recommend IVP or CT urography for those who have normal renal function, or retrograde pyelogram or MR urography for those who have renal insufficiency, and a chest radiograph every 3 to 6 months for those managed conservatively, and every 12 months for those undergoing nephroureterectomy [156].

Penile cancer

Penile cancer is the rarest of urologic malignancies, with an estimated 1470 new cases diagnosed in the United States in 2005 and approximately 270 cancer-specific deaths [1]. In patients with clinically negative inguinal lymph nodes, the strongest predictors for inguinal metastases have been shown to be primary tumor stage, grade, and the presence of lymphatic or vascular invasion [208]. There are relatively few recommendations regarding the use of imaging in the surveillance of penile carcinoma. Montie and colleagues recommended chest radiograph and inguinal CT at 3, 6, 12, and 24 months, with no

further cross-sectional imaging after 2 years if no recurrence is detected [209]. Lynch and Pettaway suggest that chest radiograph and CT of the abdomen and pelvis should be performed as clinically indicated [210]. Sanchez-Ortiz and Pettaway proposed a surveillance schedule based on risk of recurrence and initial treatment [208]. In patients treated with penile-conserving therapy or partial/total penectomy without initial inguinal lymphadenectomy, CT was recommended only in those individuals who were obese or those who have had prior inguinal surgery. Chest radiography was recommended at 12 and 24 months only in high-risk patients. For those patients who undergo initial inguinal lymphadenectomy, no imaging was recommended in those patients with negative lymph nodes. In those patients with positive lymph nodes, however, chest radiograph and CT of the abdomen, pelvis, and inguinal region were recommended every 3 months for the first 2 years, every 4 months for the third year, and every 6 months for the fourth year. Thereafter, only annual chest radiographs were recommended if no recurrence is detected. Recently, the EAU guidelines on penile cancer recommended chest radiograph and CT only for those patients found to have positive nodes on inguinal lymphadenectomy [211]. Although the EAU recommends that the intervals between examinations should be determined by each treatment center, the suggested protocol includes chest radiograph and CT every 2 to 3 months for 2 years, every 4 to 6 months during the third year, and every 6 to 12 months thereafter.

References

[1] Jemal A, Murray T, Ward E, et al. Cancer statistics, 2005. CA Cancer J Clin 2005;55:10.

[2] Cooperberg MR, Lubeck DP, Meng MV, et al. The changing face of low-risk prostate cancer: trends in clinical presentation and primary management. J Clin Oncol 2004;22:2141.

[3] Carter HB, Walsh PC, Landis P, et al. Expectant management of nonpalpable prostate cancer with curative intent: preliminary results. J Urol 2002; 167:1231.

[4] Choo R, Klotz L, Danjoux C, et al. Feasibility study: watchful waiting for localized low to intermediate grade prostate carcinoma with selective delayed intervention based on prostate specific antigen, histological and/or clinical progression. J Urol 2002;167:1664.

[5] Klotz L. Active surveillance with selective delayed intervention: using natural history to guide

treatment in good risk prostate cancer. J Urol 2004;
172:S48.

[6] Schroder FH, de Vries SH, Bangma CH. Watchful
waiting in prostate cancer: review and policy pro-
posals. BJU Int 2003;92:851.

[7] Hruby G, Choo R, Klotz L, et al. The role of serial
transrectal ultrasonography in a watchful waiting
protocol for men with localized prostate cancer.
BJU Int 2001;87:643.

[8] Messing EM, Thompson I Jr. Follow-up of conservatively managed prostate cancer: watchful waiting
and primary hormonal therapy. Urol Clin North
Am 2003;30:687.

[9] Stephenson AJ, Aprikian AG, Souhami L, et al.
Utility of PSA doubling time in follow-up of un-
treated patients with localized prostate cancer.
Urology 2002;59:652.

[10] National Comprehensive Cancer Network. National Comprehensive Cancer Network Clinical
0practice guidelines in oncology. Prostate cancer.
Version 2. Available at: http://www.nccn.org/
professionals/physician_gls/PDF/prostate.pdf.
Accessed August 5, 2005.

[11] Bill-Axelson A, Holmberg L, Ruutu M, et al. Radical prostatectomy versus watchful waiting in early
prostate cancer. N Engl J Med 2005;352:1977.

[12] Gleave MGS, Rennie P. Recent advances in prostate cancer, BPH. In: Schroeder FH, editor. Proceedings of the IV Congress on Progress and
Controversies in Oncological Urology (PACIOU
IV) New York: Parthenon Publishing; 1996.
p. 109–20.

[13] Pantelides ML, Bowman SP, George NJ. Levels of
prostate specific antigen that predict skeletal spread
in prostate cancer. Br J Urol 1992;70:299.

[14] Yap BK, Choo R, DeBoer G, et al. Are serial bone
scans useful for the follow-up of clinically localized,
low-to-intermediate–grade prostate cancer managed with watchful observation alone? BJU Int
2003;91:613.

[15] Aus G, Abbou CC, Pacik D, et al. EAU guidelines
on prostate cancer. Eur Urol 2001;40:97.

[16] Pound CR, Partin AW, Eisenberger MA, et al.
Natural history of progression after PSA elevation
following radical prostatectomy. JAMA 1999;281:
1591.

[17] Foster LS, Jajodia P, Fournier G Jr, et al. The value
of prostate specific antigen and transrectal ultrasound guided biopsy in detecting prostatic fossa recurrences following radical prostatectomy. J Urol
1993;149:1024.

[18] Nelson JB, Lepor H. Prostate cancer: radical prostatectomy. Urol Clin North Am 2003;30:703.

[19] Koppie TM, Grossfeld GD, Nudell DM, et al.
Is anastomotic biopsy necessary before radiotherapy after radical prostatectomy? J Urol
2001;166:111.

[20] Lange PH. PROSTASCINT scan for staging prostate cancer. Urology 2001;57:402.

[21] Leventis AK, Shariat SF, Kattan MW, et al. Prediction of response to salvage radiation therapy in
patients with prostate cancer recurrence after radical prostatectomy. J Clin Oncol 2001;19:1030.

[22] Nudell DM, Grossfeld GD, Weinberg VK, et al.
Radiotherapy after radical prostatectomy: treatment outcomes and failure patterns. Urology
1999;54:1049.

[23] Kagan AR, Steckel RJ. Surveillance of patients
with prostate cancer after treatment: the roles of se-
rologic and imaging studies. Med Pediatr Oncol
1993;21:327.

[24] Theodorescu D, Rabbani F, Donat SM. Follow-up
of genitourinary malignancies for the office urologist: a practical approach. Part 1: prostate and
bladder cancers. AUA Update Series 2004;23:297.

[25] Evans CP. Follow-up surveillance strategies for
genitourinary malignancies. Cancer 2002;94:2892.

[26] Cher ML, Bianco FJ Jr, Lam JS, et al. Limited role
of radionuclide bone scintigraphy in patients with
prostate specific antigen elevations after radical
prostatectomy. J Urol 1998;160:1387.

[27] Nudell DM, Wefer AE, Hricak H, et al. Imaging
for recurrent prostate cancer. Radiol Clin North
Am 2000;38:213.

[28] Kramer S, Gorich J, Gottfried HW, et al. Sensitivity of computed tomography in detecting local recurrence of prostatic carcinoma following radical
prostatectomy. Br J Radiol 1997;70:995.

[29] Seltzer MA, Barbaric Z, Belldegrun A, et al. Comparison of helical computerized tomography, positron emission tomography and monoclonal
antibody scans for evaluation of lymph node metastases in patients with prostate specific antigen relapse after treatment for localized prostate cancer.
J Urol 1999;162:1322.

[30] Silverman JM, Krebs TL. MR imaging evaluation
with a transrectal surface coil of local recurrence
of prostatic cancer in men who have undergone
radical prostatectomy. AJR Am J Roentgenol
1997;168:379.

[31] Algra PR, Bloem JL, Tissing H, et al. Detection of
vertebral metastases: comparison between MR imaging and bone scintigraphy. Radiographics 1991;
11:219.

[32] Turner JW, Hawes DR, Williams RD. Magnetic
resonance imaging for detection of prostate cancer
metastatic to bone. J Urol 1993;149:1482.

[33] Kumar R, Zhuang H, Alavi A. PET in the management of urologic malignancies. Radiol Clin North
Am 2004;42:1141.

[34] Salminen E, Hogg A, Binns D, et al. Investigations
with FDG-PET scanning in prostate cancer show
limited value for clinical practice. Acta Oncol
2002;41:425.

[35] Sanz G, Robles JE, Gimenez M, et al. Positron
emission tomography with 18fluorine-labelled
deoxyglucose: utility in localized and advanced
prostate cancer. BJU Int 1999;84:1028.

[36] Hofer C, Laubenbacher C, Block T, et al. Fluorine-18-fluorodeoxyglucose positron emission tomography is useless for the detection of local recurrence after radical prostatectomy. Eur Urol 1999;36:31.

[37] Kotzerke J, Volkmer BG, Neumaier B, et al. Carbon-11 acetate positron emission tomography can detect local recurrence of prostate cancer. Eur J Nucl Med Mol Imaging 2002;29:1380.

[38] Shvarts O, Han KR, Seltzer M, et al. Positron emission tomography in urologic oncology. Cancer Control 2002;9:335.

[39] Elgamal AA, Troychak MJ, Murphy GP. ProstaScint scan may enhance identification of prostate cancer recurrences after prostatectomy, radiation, or hormone therapy: analysis of 136 scans of 100 patients. Prostate 1998;37:261.

[40] Catton C, Milosevic M, Warde P, et al. Recurrent prostate cancer following external beam radiotherapy: follow-up strategies and management. Urol Clin North Am 2003;30:751.

[41] American Society for Therapeutic Radiology and Oncology Consensus Panel. Consensus statement: guidelines for PSA following radiation therapy. Int J Radiat Oncol Biol Phys 1997;37:1035.

[42] Cox JD, Gallagher MJ, Hammond EH, et al. Consensus statements on radiation therapy of prostate cancer: guidelines for prostate re-biopsy after radiation and for radiation therapy with rising prostate-specific antigen levels after radical prostatectomy. American Society for Therapeutic Radiology and Oncology Consensus Panel. J Clin Oncol 1999;17:1155.

[43] Albertsen PC, Hanley JA, Harlan LC, et al. The positive yield of imaging studies in the evaluation of men with newly diagnosed prostate cancer: a population based analysis. J Urol 2000;163: 1138.

[44] Sodee DB, Malguria N, Faulhaber P, et al. Multicenter ProstaScint imaging findings in 2154 patients with prostate cancer. The ProstaScint Imaging Centers. Urology 2000;56:988.

[45] Nag S, Beyer D, Friedland J, et al. American Brachytherapy Society (ABS) recommendations for transperineal permanent brachytherapy of prostate cancer. Int J Radiat Oncol Biol Phys 1999;44:789.

[46] Nag S, Bice W, DeWyngaert K, et al. The American Brachytherapy Society recommendations for permanent prostate brachytherapy postimplant dosimetric analysis. Int J Radiat Oncol Biol Phys 2000;46:221.

[47] Horwitz EM, Uzzo RG, Miller N, et al. Brachytherapy for prostate cancer: follow-up and management of treatment failures. Urol Clin North Am 2003;30:737.

[48] Shinohara K. Prostate cancer: cryotherapy. Urol Clin North Am 2003;30:725.

[49] deKernion JB. Treatment of advanced renal cell carcinoma—traditional methods and innovative approaches. J Urol 1983;130:2.

[50] Rabinovitch RA, Zelefsky MJ, Gaynor JJ, et al. Patterns of failure following surgical resection of renal cell carcinoma: implications for adjuvant local and systemic therapy. J Clin Oncol 1994;12:206.

[51] Skinner DG, Colvin RB, Vermillion CD, et al. Diagnosis and management of renal cell carcinoma. A clinical and pathologic study of 309 cases. Cancer 1971;28:1165.

[52] Gofrit ON, Shapiro A, Kovalski N, et al. Renal cell carcinoma: evaluation of the 1997 TNM system and recommendations for follow-up after surgery. Eur Urol 2001;39:669.

[53] Hafez KS, Novick AC, Campbell SC. Patterns of tumor recurrence and guidelines for follow-up after nephron sparing surgery for sporadic renal cell carcinoma. J Urol 1997;157:2067.

[54] Janzen NK, Kim HL, Figlin RA, et al. Surveillance after radical or partial nephrectomy for localized renal cell carcinoma and management of recurrent disease. Urol Clin North Am 2003;30:843.

[55] Levy DA, Slaton JW, Swanson DA, et al. Stage specific guidelines for surveillance after radical nephrectomy for local renal cell carcinoma. J Urol 1998;159:1163.

[56] Ljungberg B, Alamdari FI, Rasmuson T, et al. Follow-up guidelines for nonmetastatic renal cell carcinoma based on the occurrence of metastases after radical nephrectomy. BJU Int 1999;84:405.

[57] Sandock DS, Seftel AD, Resnick MI. A new protocol for the follow-up of renal cell carcinoma based on pathological stage. J Urol 1995;154:28.

[58] Stephenson AJ, Chetner MP, Rourke K, et al. Guidelines for the surveillance of localized renal cell carcinoma based on the patterns of relapse after nephrectomy. J Urol 2004;172:58.

[59] Cerfolio RJ, Allen MS, Deschamps C, et al. Pulmonary resection of metastatic renal cell carcinoma. Ann Thorac Surg 1994;57:339.

[60] Dineen MK, Pastore RD, Emrich LJ, et al. Results of surgical treatment of renal cell carcinoma with solitary metastasis. J Urol 1988;140:277.

[61] Pontes JE, Huben R, Novick A, et al. Salvage surgery for renal cell carcinoma. Semin Surg Oncol 1989;5:282.

[62] Stief CG, Jahne J, Hagemann JH, et al. Surgery for metachronous solitary liver metastases of renal cell carcinoma. J Urol 1997;158:375.

[63] Tanguay S, Swanson DA, Putnam JB Jr. Renal cell carcinoma metastatic to the lung: potential benefit in the combination of biological therapy and surgery. J Urol 1996;156:1586.

[64] Jayson M, Sanders H. Increased incidence of serendipitously discovered renal cell carcinoma. Urology 1998;51:203.

[65] Israel GM, Bosniak MA. Renal imaging for diagnosis and staging of renal cell carcinoma. Urol Clin North Am 2003;30:499.

[66] Lamb GW, Bromwich EJ, Vasey P, et al. Management of renal masses in patients medically

unsuitable for nephrectomy—natural history, complications, and outcome. Urology 2004;64:909.

[67] Wehle MJ, Thiel DD, Petrou SP, et al. Conservative management of incidental contrast-enhancing renal masses as safe alternative to invasive therapy. Urology 2004;64:49.

[68] Gill IS, Remer EM, Hasan WA, et al. Renal cryoablation: outcome at 3 years. J Urol 2005;173:1903.

[69] Rukstalis DB, Khorsandi M, Garcia FU, et al. Clinical experience with open renal cryoablation. Urology 2001;57:34.

[70] Matsumoto ED, Watumull L, Johnson DB, et al. The radiographic evolution of radio frequency-ablated renal tumors. J Urol 2004;172:45.

[71] McDougal WS, Gervais DA, McGovern FJ, et al. Long-term follow-up of patients with renal cell carcinoma treated with radio frequency ablation with curative intent. J Urol 2005;174:61.

[72] Frank I, Blute ML, Cheville JC, et al. A multifactorial postoperative surveillance model for patients with surgically treated clear cell renal cell carcinoma. J Urol 2003;170:2225.

[73] Uzzo RG, Novick AC. Surveillance strategies following surgery for renal cell carcinoma. In: Belldegrun A, Ritchie AWS, Figlin RA, editors. Renal and adrenal tumors: biology and management. New York: Oxford Press; 2003. p. 324.

[74] Theodorescu D, Rabbani F, Donat SM. Follow-up of genitourinary malignancies for the office urologist: a practical approach. Part 2: kidney cancer and germ cell cancer of the testis. AUA Update Series 2004;23:309.

[75] National Comprehensive Cancer Network. National Comprehensive Cancer Network clinical practice guidelines in oncology. Kidney cancer. Version 2.2005. Available at: http://www.nccn.org/professionals/physician_gls/PDF/kidney.pdf. Accessed August 5, 2005.

[76] Blacher E, Johnson DE, Haynie TP. Value of routine radionuclide bone scans in renal cell carcinoma. Urology 1985;26:432.

[77] Seaman E, Goluboff ET, Ross S, et al. Association of radionuclide bone scan and serum alkaline phosphatase in patients with metastatic renal cell carcinoma. Urology 1996;48:692.

[78] Hain SF, Maisey MN. Positron emission tomography for urological tumours. BJU Int 2003;92:159.

[79] Hoh C, Figlin R, Belldegrun A. Evaluation of renal cell carcinoma with whole body FDG PET. J Nucl Med 1996;37:141.

[80] Ramdave S, Thomas GW, Berlangieri SU, et al. Clinical role of F-18 fluorodeoxyglucose positron emission tomography for detection and management of renal cell carcinoma. J Urol 2001;166:825.

[81] Licht MR, Novick AC. Nephron sparing surgery for renal cell carcinoma. J Urol 1993;149:1.

[82] Purdue MP, Devesa SS, Sigurdson AJ, et al. International patterns and trends in testis cancer incidence. Int J Cancer 2005;115:822.

[83] Ferlay J, Bray F, Pisani P, Parkin DM. GLOBOCAN 2000: cancer incidence, mortality, and prevalence worldwide. IARC cancer base number 5. Lyon (France): IARC; 2001.

[84] Mostofi FK, Sesterhenn IA, Davis CJ. Anatomy and pathology of testis cancer. In: Coffey DS, editor. Comprehensive textbook of genitourinary oncology. 2nd edition. Philadelphia: Lippincott, Williams and Wilkins; 2000. p. 909.

[85] Fatigante L, Ducci F, Campoccia S, et al. Long-term results in patients affected by testicular seminoma treated with radiotherapy: risk of second malignancies. Tumori 2005;91:144.

[86] Ruther U, Dieckmann K, Bussar-Maatz R, et al. Second malignancies following pure seminoma. Oncology 2000;58:75.

[87] Steinfeld AD, Shore RE. Second malignancies following radiotherapy for testicular seminoma. Clin Oncol (R Coll Radiol) 1990;2:273.

[88] Travis LB, Curtis RE, Storm H, et al. Risk of second malignant neoplasms among long-term survivors of testicular cancer. J Natl Cancer Inst 1997; 89:1429.

[89] Daugaard G, Petersen PM, Rorth M. Surveillance in stage I testicular cancer. APMIS 2003;111:76.

[90] Francis R, Bower M, Brunstrom G, et al. Surveillance for stage I testicular germ cell tumours: results and cost benefit analysis of management options. Eur J Cancer 2000;36:1925.

[91] Horwich A, Peckham MJ. Surveillance after orchidectomy for clinical stage I germ-cell tumours of the testis. Prog Clin Biol Res 1988;269:471.

[92] Ramakrishnan S, Champion AE, Dorreen MS, et al. Stage I seminoma of the testis: is post-orchidectomy surveillance a safe alternative to routine postoperative radiotherapy? Clin Oncol (R Coll Radiol) 1992;4:284.

[93] von der Maase H, Specht L, Jacobsen GK, et al. Surveillance following orchidectomy for stage I seminoma of the testis. Eur J Cancer 1993;29A:1931–4.

[94] Warde P, Gospodarowicz MK, Panzarella T, et al. Long term outcome and cost in the management of stage I testicular seminoma. Can J Urol 2000;7:967.

[95] National Comprehensive Cancer Network. National Comprehensive Cancer Network clinical practice guidelines in oncology. Testicular cancer. Version 1. Available at: http://www.nccn.org/professionals/physician_gls/PDF/testicular.pdf. Accessed August 5, 2005.

[96] Laguna MP, Pizzocaro G, Klepp O, et al. EAU guidelines on testicular cancer. Eur Urol 2001;40:102.

[97] Spermon JR, Witjes JA, Kiemeney LA. Efficacy of routine follow-up after first-line treatment for testicular cancer. World J Urol 2004;22:235.

[98] Harvey ML, Geldart TR, Duell R, et al. Routine computerised tomographic scans of the thorax in surveillance of stage I testicular nonseminomatous germ cell cancer—a necessary risk? Ann Oncol 2002;13:237.

[99] Fossa SD, Aass N, Kaalhus O. Radiotherapy for testicular seminoma stage I: treatment results and long-term post-irradiation morbidity in 365 patients. Int J Radiat Oncol Biol Phys 1989;16:383.

[100] Livsey JE, Taylor B, Mobarek N, et al. Patterns of relapse following radiotherapy for stage I seminoma of the testis: implications for follow-up. Clin Oncol (R Coll Radiol) 2001;13:296.

[101] Warde P, Gospodarowicz MK, Panzarella T, et al. Stage I testicular seminoma: results of adjuvant irradiation and surveillance. J Clin Oncol 1995;13:2255.

[102] Flechon A, Bompas E, Biron P, et al. Management of postchemotherapy residual masses in advanced seminoma. J Urol 2002;168:1975.

[103] Herr HW, Sheinfeld J, Puc HS, et al. Surgery for a postchemotherapy residual mass in seminoma. J Urol 1997;157:860.

[104] De Santis M, Pont J. The role of positron emission tomography in germ cell cancer. World J Urol 2004;22:41.

[105] Ganjoo KN, Chan RJ, Sharma M, et al. Positron emission tomography scans in the evaluation of postchemotherapy residual masses in patients with seminoma. J Clin Oncol 1999;17:3457.

[106] Karapetis CS, Strickland AH, Yip D, et al. Use of fluorodeoxyglucose positron emission tomography scans in patients with advanced germ cell tumour following chemotherapy: single-centre experience with long-term follow-up. Intern Med J 2003;33:427.

[107] De Santis M, Becherer A, Bokemeyer C, et al. 2–18fluoro-deoxy-D-glucose positron emission tomography is a reliable predictor for viable tumor in postchemotherapy seminoma: an update of the prospective multicentric SEMPET trial. J Clin Oncol 2004;22:1034.

[108] Cremerius U, Effert PJ, Adam G, et al. FDG PET for detection and therapy control of metastatic germ cell tumor. J Nucl Med 1998;39:815.

[109] De Santis M, Bokemeyer C, Becherer A, et al. Predictive impact of 2–18fluoro-2-deoxy-D-glucose positron emission tomography for residual postchemotherapy masses in patients with bulky seminoma. J Clin Oncol 2001;19:3740.

[110] Hain SF, O'Doherty MJ, Timothy AR, et al. Fluorodeoxyglucose positron emission tomography in the evaluation of germ cell tumours at relapse. Br J Cancer 2000;83:863.

[111] Muller-Mattheis V, Reinhardt M, Gerharz CD, et al. Positron emission tomography with [18 F]-2-fluoro-2-deoxy-D-glucose (18FDG-PET) in diagnosis of retroperitoneal lymph node metastases of testicular tumors. Urologe A 1998;37:609.

[112] Pfannenberg AC, Oechsle K, Bokemeyer C, et al. The role of [(18)F] FDG-PET, CT/MRI and tumor marker kinetics in the evaluation of post chemotherapy residual masses in metastatic germ cell tumors—prospects for management. World J Urol 2004;22:132.

[113] Putra LJ, Lawrentschuk N, Ballok Z, et al. 18F-fluorodeoxyglucose positron emission tomography in evaluation of germ cell tumor after chemotherapy. Urology 2004;64:1202.

[114] Read G, Stenning SP, Cullen MH, et al. Medical Research Council prospective study of surveillance for stage I testicular teratoma. Medical Research Council Testicular Tumors Working Party. J Clin Oncol 1992;10:1762.

[115] Nichols CR, Timmermann R, Foster RS, et al. Neoplasms of the testis. Cancer Medicine 1997;2(140):2177.

[116] Atsu N, Eskicorapci S, Uner A, et al. A novel surveillance protocol for stage I nonseminomatous germ cell testicular tumours. BJU Int 2003;92:32.

[117] Oliver RT, Ong J, Shamash J, et al. Long-term follow-up of Anglian Germ Cell Cancer Group surveillance versus patients with stage 1 nonseminoma treated with adjuvant chemotherapy. Urology 2004;63:556.

[118] Spermon JR, Roeleveld TA, van der Poel HG, et al. Comparison of surveillance and retroperitoneal lymph node dissection in Stage I nonseminomatous germ cell tumors. Urology 2002;59:923.

[119] Donohue JP, Thornhill JA, Foster RS, et al. Stage I nonseminomatous germ-cell testicular cancer—management options and risk–benefit considerations. World J Urol 1994;12:170.

[120] Gels ME, Hoekstra HJ, Sleijfer DT, et al. Detection of recurrence in patients with clinical stage I nonseminomatous testicular germ cell tumors and consequences for further follow-up: a single-center 10-year experience. J Clin Oncol 1995;13:1188.

[121] Sharir S, Jewett MA, Sturgeon JF, et al. Progression detection of stage I nonseminomatous testis cancer on surveillance: implications for the follow-up protocol. J Urol 1999;161:472.

[122] Colls BM, Harvey VJ, Skelton L, et al. Late results of surveillance of clinical stage I nonseminoma germ cell testicular tumours: 17 years' experience in a national study in New Zealand. BJU Int 1999;83:76.

[123] Kakehi Y, Kamoto T, Kawakita M, et al. Follow-up of clinical stage I testicular cancer patients: cost and risk benefit considerations. Int J Urol 2002;9:154.

[124] Segal R, Lukka H, Klotz LH, et al. Surveillance programs for early stage non-seminomatous testicular cancer: a practice guideline. Can J Urol 2001;8:1184.

[125] Boyer MJ, Cox K, Tattersall MH, et al. Active surveillance after orchiectomy for nonseminomatous testicular germ cell tumors: late relapse may occur. Urology 1997;50:588.

[126] Freedman LS, Parkinson MC, Jones WG, et al. Histopathology in the prediction of relapse of patients with stage I testicular teratoma treated by orchidectomy alone. Lancet 1987;2:294.

[127] Nicolai N, Pizzocaro G. A surveillance study of clinical stage I nonseminomatous germ cell tumors of the testis: 10-year follow-up. J Urol 1995;154: 1045.

[128] Shahidi M, Norman AR, Dearnaley DP, et al. Late recurrence in 1263 men with testicular germ cell tumors. Multivariate analysis of risk factors and implications for management. Cancer 2002;95:520.

[129] Albers P, Siener R, Kliesch S, et al. Risk factors for relapse in clinical stage I nonseminomatous testicular germ cell tumors: results of the German Testicular Cancer Study Group Trial. J Clin Oncol 2003; 21:1505.

[130] Jewett MA, Grabowski A, McKiernan J. Management of recurrence and follow-up strategies for patients with nonseminoma testis cancer. Urol Clin North Am 2003;30:819.

[131] Weissbach L, Hartlapp JH. Adjuvant chemotherapy of metastatic stage II nonseminomatous testis tumor. J Urol 1991;146:1295.

[132] Williams SD, Stablein DM, Einhorn LH, et al. Immediate adjuvant chemotherapy versus observation with treatment at relapse in pathological stage II testicular cancer. N Engl J Med 1987;317: 1433.

[133] Gietema JA, Meinardi MT, Sleijfer DT, et al. Routine chest X-rays have no additional value in the detection of relapse during routine follow-up of patients treated with chemotherapy for disseminated nonseminomatous testicular cancer. Ann Oncol 2002;13:1616.

[134] Hendry WF, Norman AR, Dearnaley DP, et al. Metastatic nonseminomatous germ cell tumors of the testis: results of elective and salvage surgery for patients with residual retroperitoneal masses. Cancer 2002;94:1668.

[135] Stephens AW, Gonin R, Hutchins GD, et al. Positron emission tomography evaluation of residual radiographic abnormalities in postchemotherapy germ cell tumor patients. J Clin Oncol 1996;14: 1637.

[136] Kollmannsberger C, Oechsle K, Dohmen BM, et al. Prospective comparison of [18F] fluorodeoxyglucose positron emission tomography with conventional assessment by computed tomography scans and serum tumor markers for the evaluation of residual masses in patients with nonseminomatous germ cell carcinoma. Cancer 2002;94:2353.

[137] Herr HW, Sheinfeld J. Is biopsy of the contralateral testis necessary in patients with germ cell tumors? J Urol 1997;158:1331.

[138] Dieckmann KP, Loy V. The value of the biopsy of the contralateral testis in patients with testicular germ cell cancer: the recent German experience. APMIS 1998;106:13.

[139] Daugaard G, Giwercman A, Skakkebaek NE. Is biopsy of the contralateral testis necessary in patients with germ cell tumors? Editorial comment. J Urol 1997;158:1334.

[140] Csapo Z, Weissmuller J, Sigel A. Sonography in the early detection of nonpalpable second testicular tumors: a prospective study. Urologe A 1987;26:334.

[141] Haukaas S, Daehlin L, Maartmann-Moe H, et al. The long-term outcome in patients with superficial transitional cell carcinoma of the bladder: a single institutional experience. BJU Int 1999;83:957.

[142] Holmang S, Hedelin H, Anderstrom C, et al. The relationship among multiple recurrences, progression and prognosis of patients with stages Ta and T1 transitional cell cancer of the bladder followed for at least 20 years. J Urol 1995;153:1823.

[143] Holmang S, Hedelin H, Anderstrom C, et al. Longterm follow-up of a bladder carcinoma cohort: routine follow-up urography is not necessary. J Urol 1998;160:45.

[144] Oosterlinck W, Lobel B, Jakse G, et al. Guidelines on bladder cancer. Eur Urol 2002;41:105.

[145] Walzer Y, Soloway MS. Should the follow-up of patients with bladder cancer include routine excretory urography? J Urol 1983;130:672.

[146] Enver MK, Miller PD, Chinegwundoh FI. Upper tract surveillance in primary bladder cancer follow-up. BJU Int 2004;94:790.

[147] Herr HW. Tumour progression and survival in patients with T1G3 bladder tumours: 15-year outcome. Br J Urol 1997;80:762.

[148] Herr HW. Tumor progression and survival of patients with high grade, noninvasive papillary (TaG3) bladder tumors: 15-year outcome. J Urol 2000;163:60.

[149] Hession P, Flynn P, Paul N, et al. Intravenous urography in urinary tract surveillance in carcinoma of the bladder. Clin Radiol 1999;54:465.

[150] Hurle R, Losa A, Manzetti A, et al. Upper urinary tract tumors developing after treatment of superficial bladder cancer: 7-year follow-up of 591 consecutive patients. Urology 1999;53:1144.

[151] Millan-Rodriguez F, Chechile-Toniolo G, Salvador-Bayarri J, et al. Upper urinary tract tumors after primary superficial bladder tumors: prognostic factors and risk groups. J Urol 2000;164:1183.

[152] Miller EB, Eure GR, Schellhammer PF. Upper tract transitional cell carcinoma following treatment of superficial bladder cancer with BCG. Urology 1993;42:26.

[153] Herr HW, Cookson MS, Soloway SM. Upper tract tumors in patients with primary bladder cancer followed for 15 years. J Urol 1996;156:1286.

[154] Rabbani F, Perrotti M, Russo P, et al. Upper-tract tumors after an initial diagnosis of bladder cancer: argument for long-term surveillance. J Clin Oncol 2001;19:94.

[155] Smith H, Weaver D, Barjenbruch O, et al. Routine excretory urography in follow-up of superficial transitional cell carcinoma of bladder. Urology 1989;34:193.

[156] National Comprehensive Cancer Network. National Comprehensive Cancer Network clinical

practice guidelines in oncology. Bladder cancer. Available at: http://www.nccn.org/professionals/physician_gls/PDF/bladder.pdf. Accessed August 5, 2005.

[157] Greven KM, Spera JA, Solin LJ, et al. Local recurrence after cystectomy alone for bladder carcinoma. Cancer 1992;69:2767.

[158] Herr HW, Bochner BH, Dalbagni G, et al. Impact of the number of lymph nodes retrieved on outcome in patients with muscle invasive bladder cancer. J Urol 2002;167:1295.

[159] Kaplan SA, Sawczuk IS, O'Toole K, et al. Contemporary cystectomy versus preoperative radiation plus cystectomy for bladder cancer. Urology 1988;32:485.

[160] Knap MM, Lundbeck F, Overgaard J. Prognostic factors, pattern of recurrence and survival in a Danish bladder cancer cohort treated with radical cystectomy. Acta Oncol 2003;42:160.

[161] Kuroda M, Meguro N, Maeda O, et al. Stage-specific follow-up strategy after cystectomy for carcinoma of the bladder. Int J Urol 2002;9:129.

[162] Schoenberg MP, Walsh PC, Breazeale DR, et al. Local recurrence and survival following nerve sparing radical cystoprostatectomy for bladder cancer: 10-year follow-up. J Urol 1996;155:490.

[163] Slaton JW, Swanson DA, Grossman HB, et al. A stage specific approach to tumor surveillance after radical cystectomy for transitional cell carcinoma of the bladder. J Urol 1999;162:710.

[164] Stein JP, Lieskovsky G, Cote R, et al. Radical cystectomy in the treatment of invasive bladder cancer: long-term results in 1054 patients. J Clin Oncol 2001;19:666.

[165] Tefilli MV, Gheiler EL, Tiguert R, et al. Urinary diversion-related outcome in patients with pelvic recurrence after radical cystectomy for bladder cancer. Urology 1999;53:999.

[166] Visser O, Nieuwenhuijzen JA, Horenblas S. Local recurrence after cystectomy and survival of patients with bladder cancer: a population-based study in greater Amsterdam. J Urol 2005;174:97.

[167] Wishnow KI, Dmochowski R. Pelvic recurrence after radical cystectomy without preoperative radiation. J Urol 1988;140:42.

[168] Yossepowitch O, Dalbagni G, Golijanin D, et al. Orthotopic urinary diversion after cystectomy for bladder cancer: implications for cancer control and patterns of disease recurrence. J Urol 2003;169:177.

[169] Bochner BH, Montie JE, Lee CT. Follow-up strategies and management of recurrence in urologic oncology bladder cancer: invasive bladder cancer. Urol Clin North Am 2003;30:777.

[170] Schuster TG, Smith DC, Montie JE. Pelvic recurrences post cystectomy: current treatment strategies. Semin Urol Oncol 2001;19:45.

[171] Westney OL, Pisters LL, Pettaway CA, et al. Presentation, methods of diagnosis and therapy for pelvic recurrence following radical cystectomy for transitional cell carcinoma of the bladder. J Urol 1998;159:792.

[172] Ghoneim MA, el Mekresh MM, el Baz MA, et al. Radical cystectomy for carcinoma of the bladder: critical evaluation of the results in 1026 cases. J Urol 1997;158:393.

[173] Leissner J, Hohenfellner R, Thuroff JW, et al. Lymphadenectomy in patients with transitional cell carcinoma of the urinary bladder; significance for staging and prognosis. BJU Int 2000;85:817.

[174] Balaji KC, McGuire M, Grotas J, et al. Upper tract recurrences following radical cystectomy: an analysis of prognostic factors, recurrence pattern and stage at presentation. J Urol 1999;162:1603.

[175] Hastie KJ, Hamdy FC, Collins MC, et al. Upper tract tumours following cystectomy for bladder cancer. Is routine intravenous urography worthwhile? Br J Urol 1991;67:29.

[176] Kenworthy P, Tanguay S, Dinney CP. The risk of upper tract recurrence following cystectomy in patients with transitional cell carcinoma involving the distal ureter. J Urol 1996;155:501.

[177] Malkowicz SB, Skinner DG. Development of upper tract carcinoma after cystectomy for bladder carcinoma. Urology 1990;36:20.

[178] Schwartz CB, Bekirov H, Melman A. Urothelial tumors of upper tract following treatment of primary bladder transitional cell carcinoma. Urology 1992;40:509.

[179] Tsuji Y, Nakamura H, Ariyoshi A. Upper urinary tract involvement after cystectomy and ileal conduit diversion for primary bladder carcinoma. Eur Urol 1996;29:216.

[180] Huguet-Perez J, Palou J, Millan-Rodriguez F, et al. Upper tract transitional cell carcinoma following cystectomy for bladder cancer. Eur Urol 2001;40:318.

[181] Caoili EM, Cohan RH, Korobkin M, et al. Urinary tract abnormalities: initial experience with multidetector row CT urography. Radiology 2002;222:353.

[182] Sudakoff GS, Guralnick M, Langenstroer P, et al. CT urography of urinary diversions with enhanced CT digital radiography: preliminary experience. AJR Am J Roentgenol 2005;184:131.

[183] Mueller-Lisse UG, Mueller-Lisse UL, Hinterberger J, et al. Tri-phasic MDCT in the diagnosis of urothelial cancer. Eur Radiol 2003;13(S1):146.

[184] McCarthy CL, Cowan NC. Multi-detector CT urography (MD-CTU) for urothelial imaging. Radiology 2002;225:237.

[185] Caoili EM, Cohan RH, Inampudi P, et al. MDCTU of upper tract uroepithelial malignancy. AJR Am J Roentgenol 2003;180:71.

[186] Chahal R, Taylor K, Eardley I, et al. Patients at high risk for upper tract urothelial cancer: evaluation of hydronephrosis using high resolution magnetic resonance urography. J Urol 2005;174:478.

[187] Farres MT, Gattegno B, Ronco P, et al. Nonneph-rotoxic, dynamic, contrast enhanced magnetic resonance urography: use in nephrology and urology. J Urol 2000;163:1191.

[188] Klein LT, Frager D, Subramanium A, et al. Use of magnetic resonance urography. Urology 1998; 52:602.

[189] Nolte-Ernsting CC, Bucker A, Adam GB, et al. Gadolinium-enhanced excretory MR urography after low-dose diuretic injection: comparison with conventional excretory urography. Radiology 1998;209:147.

[190] Nolte-Ernsting CC, Adam GB, Gunther RW. MR urography: examination techniques and clinical applications. Eur Radiol 2001;11:355.

[191] Nawfel RD, Judy PF, Schleipman AR, et al. Patient radiation dose at CT urography and conventional urography. Radiology 2004;232:126.

[192] Heicappell R, Muller-Mattheis V, Reinhardt M, et al. Staging of pelvic lymph nodes in neoplasms of the bladder and prostate by positron emission tomography with 2-[(18)F]-2-deoxy-D-glucose. Eur Urol 1999;36:582.

[193] Kosuda S, Kison PV, Greenough R, et al. Preliminary assessment of fluorine-18 fluorodeoxyglucose positron emission tomography in patients with bladder cancer. Eur J Nucl Med 1997;24:615.

[194] de Jong IJ, Pruim J, Elsinga PH, et al. Visualisation of bladder cancer using (11)C-choline PET: first clinical experience. Eur J Nucl Med Mol Imaging 2002;29:1283.

[195] Canfield SE, Dinney CP, Droller MJ. Surveillance and management of recurrence for upper tract transitional cell carcinoma. Urol Clin North Am 2003; 30:791.

[196] Cozad SC, Smalley SR, Austenfeld M, et al. Transitional cell carcinoma of the renal pelvis or ureter: patterns of failure. Urology 1995;46:796.

[197] Deligne E, Colombel M, Badet L, et al. Conservative management of upper urinary tract tumors. Eur Urol 2002;42:43.

[198] Elliott DS, Segura JW, Lightner D, et al. Is nephroureterectomy necessary in all cases of upper tract transitional cell carcinoma? Long-term results of conservative endourologic management of upper tract transitional cell carcinoma in individuals with a normal contralateral kidney. Urology 2001;58:174.

[199] Hall MC, Womack S, Sagalowsky AI, et al. Prognostic factors, recurrence, and survival in transitional cell carcinoma of the upper urinary tract: a 30-year experience in 252 patients. Urology 1998;52:594.

[200] Jabbour ME, Smith AD. Primary percutaneous approach to upper urinary tract transitional cell carcinoma. Urol Clin North Am 2000;27:739.

[201] Kang CH, Yu TJ, Hsieh HH, et al. The development of bladder tumors and contralateral upper urinary tract tumors after primary transitional cell carcinoma of the upper urinary tract. Cancer 2003;98:1620.

[202] Keeley FX Jr, Bibbo M, Bagley DH. Ureteroscopic treatment and surveillance of upper urinary tract transitional cell carcinoma. J Urol 1997;157: 1560.

[203] Munoz VD, Rebassa LM, Hidalgo PF, et al. Upper urinary tract tumors: results of treatment and follow-up. Arch Esp Urol 1999;52:333.

[204] Chen GL, El Gabry EA, Bagley DH. Surveillance of upper urinary tract transitional cell carcinoma: the role of ureteroscopy, retrograde pyelography, cytology and urinalysis. J Urol 2000;164:1901.

[205] Oosterlinck W, Solsona E, van der Meijden AP, et al. EAU guidelines on diagnosis and treatment of upper urinary tract transitional cell carcinoma. Eur Urol 2004;46:147.

[206] Razdan S, Johannes J, Cox M, et al. Current practice patterns in urologic management of upper-tract transitional-cell carcinoma. J Endourol 2005;19:366.

[207] Hisataki T, Miyao N, Masumori N, et al. Risk factors for the development of bladder cancer after upper tract urothelial cancer. Urology 2000; 55:663.

[208] Sanchez-Ortiz RF, Pettaway CA. Natural history, management, and surveillance of recurrent squamous cell penile carcinoma: a risk-based approach. Urol Clin North Am 2003;30:853.

[209] Montie JE. Follow-up after penectomy for penile cancer. Urol Clin North Am 1994;21:725.

[210] Lynch D, Pettaway C. Tumors of the penis. In: Walsh P, Retik A, Vaughan E, et al, editors. Campbell's urology. 8th edition. Philadelphia: W.B. Saunders; 2002. p. 2945.

[211] Solsona E, Algaba F, Horenblas S, et al. EAU guidelines on penile cancer. Eur Urol 2004;46:1.

**ELSEVIER
SAUNDERS**

Urol Clin N Am 33 (2006) 397–408

**UROLOGIC
CLINICS
of North America**

New Technology for Imaging and Documenting Urologic Procedures

Charles G. Marguet, MD, W. Patrick Springhart, MD,
Glenn M. Preminger, MD*

*The Comprehensive Kidney Stone Center, The Division of Urology, Department of Surgery,
Duke University Medical Center, Box 3167, Room 1572 D, White Zone, Durham, NC 27710, USA*

Adequate exposure is paramount to the success of any surgical procedure. During open surgical intervention, the choice of incision and retraction dictates the quality of exposure. Endo–urologic and laparoscopic procedures, however, are dependent upon high-quality optics, which provide the surgeon the exposure necessary for successful intervention. For this reason, much of this article focuses on imaging, with particular emphasis on newer digital cameras and monitor technology.

Previously, the ability to capture, manipulate, and document surgical procedures tended to be cumbersome and complex. Yet, the ability to document the procedure is essential for educating and training resident and postgraduate urologists. To this end, the technologic capacity to reproduce video and still images in digital or analog form remains a challenge. Future developments will be instrumental in allowing for more user-friendly interfaces. This article addresses many of these issues.

The original design and construction of most operating rooms occurred without the minimally invasive, endoscopic approach in mind. That is, most current operating rooms were designed for open surgery. As a consequence, adjustments were made to accommodate laparoscopic and minimally invasive technology. Recent operating room designs recognize the fundamental differences between open and laparoscopic surgery. Thus, specialized rooms are being developed that are much more conducive to consistent and trouble-free documentation of urologic procedures.

Digital imaging

Numerous recent major improvements have enhanced video endoscopic surgery greatly [1–3], specifically, the development of how optical information is captured, transmitted, and produced as an image. Initially, an optical image is converted to an electronic signal [3]. This electronic information, which includes color and light (luminance), is transmitted to a video monitor, where it is scanned to produce an image on the screen.

The Standard National Television Systems Committee (NTSC) video signal uses a limited bandwidth that includes the color and luminance information in a single or composite signal. Obstacles with this format include signal noise, caused by the camera having to first process color and luminance information separately and then combining both segments of information to create a video signal. This video noise or cross-talk may be the cause of decreased resolution, resulting in grainy images and a loss of information around the edges of the video image. Furthermore, this video noise will amplify as additional copies of the video signal are reproduced.

Since the introduction of digital imaging, two newer video formats have been introduced [4]. The first format, called Y/C (Y = luminescence, C = color), is a component signal that allows the color and luminance information to be carried as two separate signals. This component video signal, also known as superVHS (or S-VHS), contains less cross-talk and therefore appears

* Corresponding author.

E-mail address: glenn.preminger@duke.edu
(G.M. Preminger).

urologic.theclinics.com

cleaner and sharper than images generated by composite signals. Similar to the NTSC format, the video signal in the Y/C format is carried by a single cable, although the color information and luminance information remain separated.

The second digital video format is known as RGB (red-green-blue). This format is also a component signal. In contrast to the Y/C format, however, the video information (color and luminance) is separated into four signals: red, green, blue, and a timing signal. Additionally, each signal carries its own luminance information, requiring four separate cables (red-green-blue, and sync) in contrast to NTSC and Y/C. The separation of each video signal is performed electronically in the camera head. In contradistinction to the NTSC or Y/C format, the RGB format requires less electronic processing, because the color information and luminance information are separate from the onset. Thus, the RGB image quality is enhanced greatly compared with the other two formats. Although most video monitors will accept standard NTSC video formats, a special (and more expensive) monitor is required to accept Y/C and RGB formats. Despite the increased cost, superior image quality will result when compared with the standard NTSC format.

Images and signals in the NTSC format (standard analog) are processed as voltages (Fig. 1 A). It is therefore inevitable that small errors in recording and reproducing these voltages accumulate with each generation of the video image. As a result, multiple copies of an analog image will reveal a decrease in the quality of the video pictures. Conversely, a digital converter will change all video signals into precise numbers (eg, 0 or 1) in the digital video formats (Y/C and RGB) (Fig. 1 B). Conversion to a digital signal gives the video image immunity to noise buildup or image quality degradation. In addition, image processing can be performed to enhance or alter the digital video images. Once the video information has been digitized, it can be merged with other formats, such as text or audio data, and manipulated without any loss of information.

Video endoscopy

The development of the digital video endoscope has been a major advance in endoscopic systems. The ability to miniaturize chip technology led to the development and incorporation of the charged coupled device (CCD) chip into the distal end of an endoscope (chip on a stick or EndoEye, Olympus America, Melville, NY) (Fig. 2). Previously, optical images from the distal end of the scope relied on the transmission of that image through an internal optical conduit, such as fiber optics, to the proximal end of the scope where the camera was attached to the eyepiece. CCD technology allows the image to be focused

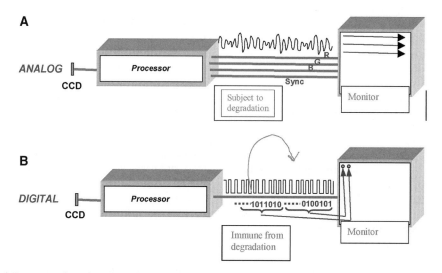

Fig. 1. (*A*) Representation of analog video imaging in which video signals remain as voltage waveforms. Charged coupled device (CCD). (*B*) In contrast, digital video systems convert the analog video information to a digital format, which must be converted back to analog information before it is viewed on the video monitor. Conversion to a digital signal gives the digital video image immunity to noise buildup or image quality degradation.

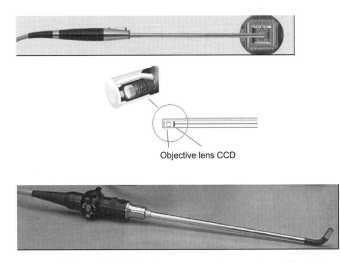

Objective lens CCD

Fig. 2. Chip on a stick or EndoEye technology. This technological advance allowed for the development of the flexible laparoscope. (*From* Olympus America, Melville, New York.)

on and immediately captured by the CCD chip, whereupon it is digitized and converted into electrical signals for transmission. This design has the benefit of fewer interfaces, allowing the digital information to be transmitted directly to an image display unit with minimal image loss, interference, and distortion [5,6] (Fig. 3). As internal optics are not required in the long and flexible shafts of these instruments, durable deflection mechanisms can be used for the first time in laparoscopy and to improve the durability of flexible endoscopes [7–9]. Additionally, because the signal can be transmitted without the need to attach the camera head to the eyepiece of the scope, the videoscope signal can be incorporated into the light cord cable for attachment to the video system. This provides for a more lightweight and convenient setup. This technology has been incorporated into larger, rigid endoscopes (laparoscopes) and some flexible endoscopes (colonoscopes, bronchoscopes, and cystoscopes) [4,10,11]. One can expect to see such an integrated digital videoendoscope replacing smaller caliber ureteroscopes and cystoscopes in the near future [12].

An additional development in digital camera technology includes the use of a single monochrome CCD chip with alternating red, green, and blue illumination to form a color image rather than using three chips with three separate color filters. This application allows further reduction in space requirements, while taking advantage of high-resolution monochrome CCD chip technology [5]. This design is used in a digital

videocystoscope (Olympus America, Mellville, New York). One can expect similar technologic innovations to be incorporated into digital laparoscopes also.

Digital imaging, video documentation, and editing

Digital imaging is revolutionizing the field of videoendoscopy. Despite the initial acquisition of image signal in the analog format, technologic advances allow conversion to digital format through a digital camera or scanner. Furthermore, the introduction of digital still cameras allows image documentation and editing to exist at a higher level. As a consequence, newer surgical video systems have integrated a digital image capture system that allows the immediate capturing of still images from endoscopic procedures [8] (Fig. 4). A less expensive alternative is the digital still image capture adapter, which can be connected to endoscopic camera systems [13]. Digital still images usually can be recorded in JPEG (.jpg-Joint Photographic Experts Group), TIFF (.tif-tagged image file format) or BMP (.bmp-bitmap) formats. Using various computer software packages, these images may be incorporated into the patient's medical record and used for the creation of an image library for the enhancement of one's practice [14,15]. Fortunately, the digital images may be stored in different formats depending on the quality of image needed for editing. In cases where storage is not an issue, the image should be obtained at its highest resolution. This process

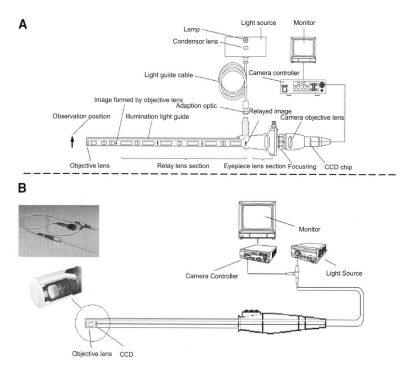

Fig. 3. (*A*) Traditional rod and lens technology. (*B*) Videoscope technology. (*From* Olympus America, Melville, New York.)

allows future use of the highest caliber of image, or conversion of the image to a differing format, without the loss of quality. For instance, low-resolution images, in the range of 1 to 2 megapixels, can be used for E-mail attachments or Power

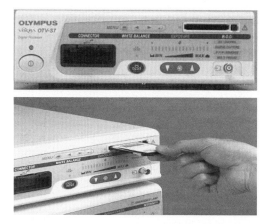

Fig. 4. Still images and short video clips (depending on resolution) can be captured on a digital card. Direct digital video stream can be captured on a computer, digital camcorder, or digital recorder by means of an IEEE 1394 fire wire connector on the back panel. (*From* Olympus America, Melville, New York.)

Point presentations. Printed images require a higher quality image between 3 to 4 megapixels. In the past, most video recordings during endoscopic procedures were performed with conventional analog formats, such as VHS or SVHS, which could be digitally converted. Now, with the advent of digital video recording devices, video footage can be recorded directly into a digital format (ie, DV [digital video], MPEG [Moving Picture Experts Group] and AVI [audio video interleave]) (Fig. 5). These video capturing systems can be part of an expensive commercial integrated video system, DV camera, DVD recorder, or a low cost personal computer with digital video capture card [16]. Moreover, digital video editing may be performed on a personal computer using various video editing software (eg, Adobe Premiere, Adobe Systems Incorporated, San Jose, California; Windows Movie Maker, Microsoft Corporation, Redmond, Washington).

Miniaturization of storage devices has resulted in the ability to store smaller still digital images onto more portable digital storage media (eg, SmartMedia, Toshiba Corp., Tokyo, Japan; Compact Flash, ScanDisk Corp., Sunnyvale, CA; Secure Digital; Multi Media card; and Memory Stick, Sony Corp., Tokyo, Japan) up to

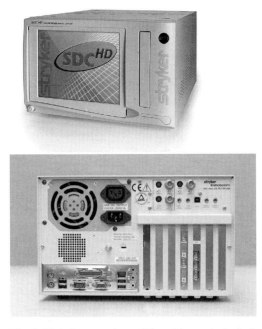

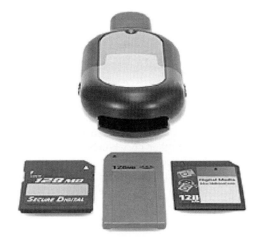

Fig. 6. Miniaturization of storage devices has resulted in the ability to store smaller still digital images onto more portable digital storage media.

Fig. 5. Digital capture is possible and increasingly flexible, offering the ability to store directly to DVD in all forms of MPEG or AVI. Hand devices offer Ethernet connectivity, providing video conferencing capability. Video capture directly to an 80 GB hard drive is possible, as is streaming to computer or video camera by means of SVIDEO, IEEE-1394, Serial port. (*From* Stryker Endoscopy, San Jose, California.)

1 gigabyte. For larger files especially, video clips, Zip Disk (up to 750 megabytes [MB]), CD-ROM (up to 700 MB), and lately DVD (up to 17GB) can be used (Fig. 6). Also, with the introduction of portable hard drives, the ability to store over 300 GB of information is available. Image storage, however, continues to pose a challenge, especially with large volumes of digital files performed on the institutional level. Picture archiving and communication systems (PACS) are being implemented to eventually replace the need for hard copy films in medical imaging [17–19].

Video light sources

Additional advances in imaging have been a result from the use of a high-intensity light source, generated from either halogen or xenon sources. The ability to adjust light intensity using several mechanisms has been a recent advancement. For example, certain light sources have an automatic light-sensing feature that quickly adjusts the light output as required by the camera. This feature becomes particularly relevant as the endoscope moves through areas of differing volumes, such as the transition from the urethra into the bladder, where a greater amount of light intensity is needed. In effect, the light intensity will adjust automatically to maintain a preselected illumination level. Alternatively, some camera systems are equipped with an automatic iris system, similar to the human eye, which will electronically increase or decrease the aperture of the camera. Obviously, if the camera system is equipped with such a light-sensing feature, there is no need for an automatic light-adjusting light source.

Newer CCDs or image sensor-based endoscopic cameras feature electronic exposure. The mechanism of this system works by varying the light gathering time interval, or exposure period, of the CCD as the image is captured. Typical CCD exposure periods range from approximately 1/60 of a second to 1/10000 of a second under very bright conditions. This is an additional mechanism to maintain the brightness of an image. When the image brightness must be reduced to improve picture clarity, the image signal exposure period can be reduced electronically instead of adjusting the iris of the light source.

The role of shadows and their importance in depth perception and spatial orientation have been established. Studies have demonstrated that endoscopic task performance significantly improves with video systems that provide proper illumination and appropriate shadows in the operative field [20]. Currently, many endoscopes employ a simple frontal illumination technique that produces an optically flat and shadowless image. This results in an image with poor contrast. Recent innovations in illumination technology use single-point or multi-point shadow-inducing systems. For instance, one of these techniques employs the use of two independent illumination fiber bundles, with one fiber bundle ending at the front lens, as designed in conventional endoscopes, and the other fiber bundle ending behind the tip of endoscope. Because of the formation of shadows, spatial orientation and perception between anatomical structures are enhanced considerably [21].

Image transmission

Technologic advances continue to emerge in the form of data transmission, storage, and display. As a result, the ability now exists to perform these functions from a workstation in the office, hospital, or even from a remote off-site location. One limitation to the efficiency of this process is the narrow bandwidth of standard telephone lines. In simplistic terms, bandwidth refers to the capacity of information that can be transmitted in a unit of time (eg, bits per second or bps). To this end, conduits of data transfer with a narrow bandwidth, such as telephone lines, restrict data transmission, whereas conduits with wider bandwidths, such as fiberoptic lines, enhance data transmission, Thus, attempting to transmit data files containing high-resolution images or full-motion video over narrow bandwidth conduits may result in the delay or loss of data, resulting in poorer resolution images, or video files that play at intermittent sequences. Additional modes of image transmission are used in the communications industry and may be applied to the medical workplace.

Fiberoptic cable

Fiberoptic cable has the ability to transmit significantly more information than standard coaxial copper cable, and thus supplants it. For instance, one fiberoptic fiber can carry upwards of 1.7 gigabytes per second. This rate is thousands of times faster than data transmitted over standard coaxial cable. Because of the physical properties of image transference, optical fiber has a lower attenuation than coaxial cable and is not subject to electromagnetic interference.

The major advantage of fiberoptics is that large amounts of digitized information (eg, video,

audio, or data) can be transmitted rapidly [22]. This increased speed of transmission is especially important when dealing with the large amount of digital information contained in video images. Notwithstanding the prevalence of copper cable, it is implicit that the overall advantages of fiberoptic conduits eventually will cause it to become the primary mode of transmitting voice and data information.

Wireless local area network

Recently, wireless local area networks (LAN) also known as WiFi, have been introduced in the health care setting. Using electromagnetic waves, typically in the frequency of 2.4 GHz, these networks allow wireless devices to communicate with one another through access points or antennae. This allows a physician to receive data and images regarding patient care throughout a hospital. Similar to cordless telephones, these WiFi devices have a certain range of 100 to 300 m, within which they should be operated. The standards and specifications of wireless LAN are created by the Institute of Electrical and Electronics Engineers (IEEE). The original WiFi, or 802.11 b, allowed the transmission of data at a rate of 11 megabits per second. Currently, however, the standard is the 802.11 g, and provides for wireless data transmission at speeds up to 54 megabits per second. At these transmission rates, digital still and video image transmission becomes practical [23].

The advantages of a wireless network are, as the name implies, the lack of having to install a wired network and the ability to communicate with mobile users. Initial setup costs and the potential need for battery requirements at mobile workstations can be a shortcoming for installment. The interference of wireless devices with medical devices also has been a concern. Yet, interference has been shown to occur only when the medical device was within 10 cm of the LAN transmitter [24]. Wireless networks have been used successfully to transmit radiographic images for interpretation, and to transmit a live broadcast of a laparoscopic surgery to handheld computers for instructional purposes [25,26].

Satellite communications

Wireless local area networks and fiberoptic conduits can provide data transference localized to areas accessed by each respective technology. Remote areas devoid of antennae for receiving an electromagnetic signal of WiFi or lacking fiberoptic cable lines are at a disadvantage, however. Despite this, the use of satellite communications has allowed the transmission of digitized video images to remote areas that are not linked by coaxial cable or fiberoptic conduit. Furthermore, satellite communications currently allow the performance of teleconferencing and telemedicine, where voice and video images can be transmitted to remote sites almost instantaneously. Combinations of fiberoptic cable and satellite transmission systems may one day link distant operating rooms to major medical centers, and thereby facilitate the performance and teaching of advanced endoscopic procedures. Also, instead of a surgeon traveling long distances to assist and proctor in remote areas, they can guide other surgeons, through telepresence surgery, from a central site.

Video system set-up

Video cart

The video cart is an integral component for the entire video capturing system that allows one to easily transport the documentation system from one surgical suite to another (Fig. 7). The video cart should have the capacity to hold video camera electronics, a light source, and various recording devices such as a VCR, printer, or video disc recorder. Moreover, some video carts also will have room to hold the laparoscopic insufflator and electrocautery units. Particular attention also should focus on the capability of the cart to hold carbon dioxide tanks that will be used during laparoscopy. Lastly, one should be able to adequately secure the cart during storage to prevent equipment loss.

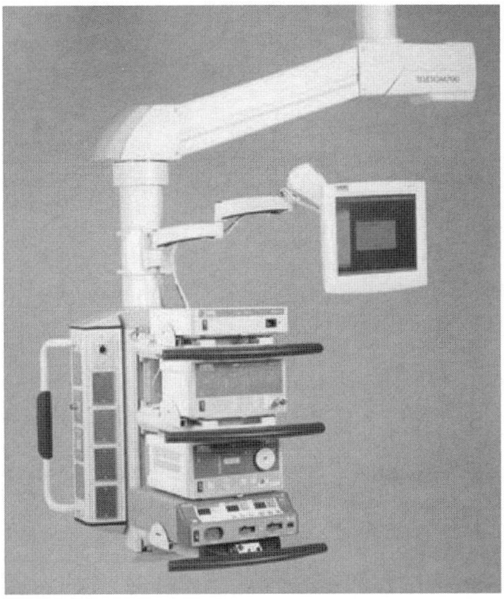

Video set-up

The authors' conventional operating room set-up places the video cart, containing equipment pertinent to the individual procedure, directly across from the operating surgeon. A second high-resolution video monitor will be placed on the other side of the table to be used by the assistants. If only one video monitor is available, it should be placed directly at the end of the operating table so that both the surgeon and assistant may view it. Recently, with the construction of an endoscopic suite, all endoscopic procedures at the authors' institution are performed entirely off the video monitor(s).

In the past, endoscopic surgeons relied on mobile video carts to be transported to their assigned rooms. A fundamental difference in

Fig. 7. Video carts (wheeled or suspended, as shown here) contain video camera electronics, light source, and various recording devices.

equipment needs and room orientation, however, has been recognized between open and endoscopic surgery. Consequently, specialized rooms are being constructed to provide items such as dedicated carbon dioxide lines to obviate the need to change tanks during an operation. Occupational hazards, such as musculoskeletal strain, may be related to suboptimal operating room design. Studies have demonstrated significant stressors to the surgeon induced by laparoscopy. Many of these stressors are related to monitor placement, camera holding, trocar placement, and table position and height [27–30]. Additional features, such as ceiling-mounted monitors allow for improving the ergonomics surrounding minimally invasive urologic procedures (Fig. 8). As of yet, no prospective study has been undertaken to determine the effects of these specially designed operating rooms on musculoskeletal complications. Some studies, however, suggest that muscle fatigue is related to the poor ergonometric characteristics of some operating rooms and that attempts to improve the ergonomics may improve overall operating room efficiency [31,32].

Three-dimensional video endoscopic/laparoscopic systems

In addition to adequate exposure, stereoscopic vision is paramount for precise surgical

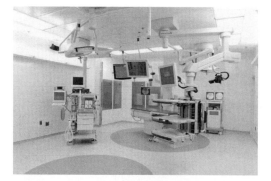

Fig. 8. Current (future) endoscopic/laparoscopic operating room. Ceiling mounted flat panel monitors. Built-in endoscopy table with adequate room for laparoscopic applications. Ceiling mounted camera for external footage. Touch panel control allowing for routing of different source images on different monitors. Wall plug in for C-arm integration with room monitors. Wall panel integrating operating room with audiovisual center allowing for video capture, integration with conference rooms, and teleconferencing. (*From* Duke University Medical Center, Durham, North Carolina.)

performance during laparoscopic and endoscopic surgery. Most current video endoscopic systems provide a two-dimensional, flat image to the operating surgeon. Yet, recent advances in imaging technology allow three-dimensional video techniques to be used during laparoscopic surgery (Fig. 9).

Four basic principles of stereoendoscopic image processing are present in most three-dimensional video systems: presentation of left and right images on a single monitor, image capture, conversion of 60 to 120 Hz images, and separation of the left and right eyes images [24,33]. A three-dimensional system uses two images from the operating field, similar to human eyes, which are transmitted and displayed on the monitor. In doing so, the images of the right and left cameras are alternated rapidly at a frequency of 100/120 Hz to display the three-dimensional image. This method also is known as sequential display procedure. Several image-capturing methods have been employed, including the dual-lens system, single-lens systems, the electronic videoendoscopic system, and a system of single rod-lenses with two beam paths. Displaying a three-dimensional image may be accomplished with either active liquid crystal display glasses or polarizing glasses. In both cases, the brain fuses the right- and left-sided images on the appropriate imaging site, and in effect simulates depth. Based on the physiology of

retinal image persistence, this technology is quite different from normal stereoscopic imaging, wherein the two independent images are shown to both eyes simultaneously [34]. An additional mechanism of three-dimensional imaging is created by mimicking the human eye's acquisition of images, that is, the presentation of two independent images to each eye. The daVinci robotic system (Intuitive Surgical, Sunnyvale, California), featuring a fixed, head-mounted display, uses this technology.

Comparisons of two- and three-dimensional video systems have offered conflicting results in experimental and clinical practice. Because of the high cost and lack of availability, three-dimensional systems are not used widely. Furthermore, studies have suggested a lack of improved performance from a three-dimensional system and that it may be more advantageous to have a higher-resolution video system than three-dimensional endoscopic image [35–37]. The vast majority of three-dimensional imaging system use is during laparoscopic, robotic surgical procedures, for true stereoscopic imaging [38–40]. Additional prospective studies are needed to compare surgical efficiency and surgeon fatigability from both systems.

Virtual reality

Practitioners of any vocation require certain skill sets, and endoscopic surgeons are no exception. Yet, there often are reduced training opportunities available to trainees because of the expense, supply, and ethical dilemmas surrounding animal or cadaveric models [41–43]. The ability to gain certain basic skill sets from laboratory models exists for beginners in laparoscopy; however, these skills may not be sufficient to the various clinical scenarios that exist [44]. Additionally, inanimate simulators lack the tactile feedback available from the living model.

Technologic advances in virtual reality simulation (VR) allow an interactive environment that simulates through a dynamic, realistic environment. Furthermore, VR circumvents the moral and ethical dilemmas associated with patients and animal models. Advances in computer software have allowed VR simulators to more accurately reproduce real-life anatomy. The prototypical simulator should, as in endoscopic surgery, provide two- or three-dimensional spatial cues, shadowing, and tactile feedback.

Earlier simulators provided a simplistic experience for endoscopic procedures such as

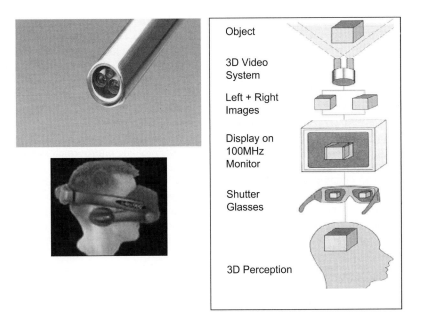

Fig. 9. Three-dimensional stereoendoscope. Schematic diagram of three-dimensional video imaging system. The two images are projected on a screen, and the glasses bring the two together, giving the impression of a three-dimensional image. Alternatively, the separate images can be presented separately to the left and right eye through a head set. This is currently available as part of the DaVinci robotic system and theoretically can be developed by means of a head-mounted display. (*From* www.stereo3d.com, Christoph Bungert, Koenigstein, Germany.)

ureteroscopy, but lacked true anatomic representation and featured inadequate computer graphics [41,42,45]. Subsequent advances in computing power and VR graphics have resulted in more advance simulators (eg, URO Mentor system, Symbionix, Tel Aviv, Israel). This VR endoscopic simulator not only provides more realistic anatomic projections, but places simulations of most urologic procedures in the urologist's hands. For instance, cystoscopy and retrograde pyelograms are simulated using a simulated real-time fluoroscopic unit. Additionally, simulation of ureteric access and endoscopic procedures are provided, including guide wire placement and stone fragmentation and removal. Additionally, studies have demonstrated a more rapid acquisition and translation of skills by those in urologic training when using these simulators [46–49]. Not only can trainees be taught novel skills using VR simulation, but these skills can be tested and validated. Studies have demonstrated that endoscopic simulation can decrease the learning curve in routine and complex procedures [43,50]. Because of additional software and computer upgrades, VR simulation also has become more life-like in the simulation of laparoscopic surgery [51–54]. Some day, one may expect not only to have written and verbal examinations to assess ones competency, but also a skill assessment using VR demonstration.

Internet and telemedicine

The combination of electronic and communication advancements has allowed patient care to sometimes take place from a remote location. Telemedicine (defined as patient care from a remote location) has become a feasible part of patient care. Advances in digital imaging, high-speed computer connections, and the widespread availability of the Internet have allowed a steady growth of telemedicine within urology [55]. Digital image formats, from simple digital camera images to complex images of MRI may be transmitted over the Internet. Transmission speed varies from 128 kilobits per second (kbps) using an integrated services digital network (ISDN) line, 1.54 megabits per second (Mbps) using a T1 line, 6 Mbps using a coaxial line, and into the gigabits per second (Gbps) using optical fiber lines [13,14,56]. Two variations of telemedicine exist. The first is synchronous and real-time video conferencing. In general, real-time motion requires that images are generated at a speed of 30 frames per second [57]. The advantage of live video teleconferencing is that it allows real-time interaction between physicians and patients with full motion audio-visual images, developing a true physician–patient relationship. In addition, various medical centers can be linked with the teleconferencing facility to promote tele-education and teleconsultation. With proper equipment, digital images, including endoscopic pictures, pathologic slides, and radiographic images also can be transmitted in real time. The cost of real-time telemedicine systems and communication networks has prohibited its widespread use. As an example, some teleconferencing systems can cost more than $80,000, not including connection fees that may be as high as $800 per month [58]. Studies have demonstrated that one could provide high-quality high-definition television image-orientated telemedicine by means of ISDN lines or communication satellites. The minimum set-up cost is significant, however, at greater than $1,000,000 [59].

A second variation of telemedicine exists using an asynchronous or store and forward system, whereby the information is transmitted by means of E-mail or the Internet. At his or her own convenience, the recipient may review, respond, and store the data transmitted. Current asynchronous technology also is improving with better software development, resulting in a more secure transmission of encrypted data over the Internet [14]. Notwithstanding the lack of a real-time interaction, asynchronous telemedicine remains efficacious in medical care and training [56].

There is a lack of standardization for image data exchange in telemedicine. One such input format, Digital Imaging and Communications in Medicine, exists. No standard exists for other digital images such as video clips or still images. Consequently, there is a need for the future standardization and integration of telemedicine hardware [59].

Additional challenges for telemedicine include standardization of physician licensing, regulation of telemedicine, patient confidentiality issues, and reimbursement for consultations.

Laparoscopic applications

Today, telemedicine, and specifically telesurgery, has arrived. Kavoussi and colleagues proved the concept when they published their initial laboratory experience with telerobotic-assisted laparoscopic surgery [60–65]. On the other side of the globe, telesurgery has taken place. In Rome, where at the time laparoscopic surgery had been recently introduced, five patients underwent laparoscopic surgery while surgeons in Baltimore proctored the procedures in real time [66]. The telemedicine and telesurgical approach may afford improved patient care by allowing highly experienced surgeons to either perform or participate in the more recent and advanced endoscopic and laparoscopic procedures.

Technologic improvements in communication, computer processing, image graphics, and operating room ergonomics will continue to evolve. As the costs of telemedicine decrease, greater use of telemedicine should occur. These technical improvements also will result in improvements in the training and the performance of endo–urologic and laparoscopic procedures [60,65,67,68].

References

[1] Kennedy TJ, Preminger GM. Impact of video on endourology. J Endourol 1987;1:75.

[2] Litwiler SE, Preminger GM. Advances in electronic imaging for laparoscopy. J Endourol 1993;7:S195.

[3] Preminger GM. Video-assisted transurethral resection of the prostate. J Endourol 1991;5:161.

[4] Knyrim K, Seidlitz H, Vakil N, et al. Perspectives in electronic endoscopy. Past, present, and future of fibers and CCDs in medical endoscopes. Endoscopy 1990;22(Suppl 1):2.

[5] Boppart SA, Deutsch TF, Rattner DW. Optical imaging technology in minimally invasive surgery. Current status and future directions. Surg Endosc 1999; 13:718.

[6] Cuschieri A. Technology for minimal access surgery. Interview by Judy Jones. BMJ 1999;319:1304.

[7] Afane JS, Olweny EO, Bercowsky E, et al. Flexible ureteroscopes: a single center evaluation of the durability and function of the new endoscopes smaller than 9Fr. J Urol 2000;164:1164.

[8] Auge BK, Preminger GM. Digital cameras and documentation in urologic practice. AUA update series XXI. Linthicum (MD): American Urologic Association Press; 2002.

[9] Levisohn PM. Safety and tolerability of topiramate in children. J Child Neurol 2000;15(Suppl 1):S22.

[10] Niwa H, Kawaguchi A, Miyahara T, et al. Clinical use of new video endoscopes (EVIS 100 and 200). Endoscopy 1992;24:222.

[11] Pelosi MA, Kadar N, Pelosi MA III. The electronic video operative laparoscope. J Am Assoc Gynecol Laparosc 1993;1:54.

[12] Springhart WP, Maloney MM, Sur RL, et al. Digital video ureteroscope: a new paradigm in ureteroscopy. J Urol 2005;173:428S.

[13] Kuo RL, Preminger GM. Current urologic applications of digital imaging. J Endourol 2001;15:53.

[14] Kuo RL, Aslan P, Dinlenc CZ, et al. Secure transmission of urologic images and records over the Internet. J Endourol 1999;13:141.

[15] Kuo RL, Delvecchio FC, Preminger GM. Use of a digital camera in the urologic setting. Urology 1999;53:613.

[16] Wurnig PN, Hollaus PH, Wurnig CH, et al. A new method for digital video documentation in surgical procedures and minimally invasive surgery. Surg Endosc 2003;17:232.

[17] Arernso RL, Andriole KP, Avrin DE, et al. Computers in imaging and health care: now and in the future. J Digit Imaging 2000;13:145.

[18] Fujino MA, Ikeda M, Yamamoto Y, et al. Development of an integrated filing system for endoscopic images. Endoscopy 1991;23:11.

[19] Martinez R, Cole C, Rozenblit J, et al. Common object request broker architecture (CORBA)-based security services for the virtual radiology environment. J Digit Imaging 2000;13:59.

[20] Emam TA, Hanna G, Cuschieri A. Ergonomic principles of task alignment, visual display, and direction of execution of laparoscopic bowel suturing. Surg Endosc 2002;16:267.

[21] Schurr MO, Kunert W, Arezzo A, et al. The role and future of endoscopic imaging systems. Endoscopy 1999;31:557.

[22] Huang H. Image storage, transmission, and manipulation. Minim Invasive Ther Allied Technol 1992; 1:85.

[23] Yoshihiro A, Nakata N, Harada J, et al. Wireless local area networking for linking a PC reporting system and PACS: clinical feasibility in emergency reporting. Radiographics 2002;22:721.

[24] Tan YH, Preminger GM. Advances in video and imaging in ureteroscopy. Urol Clin North Am 2004;31:33.

[25] Gandsas A, McIntire K, Park A. Live broadcast of laparoscopic surgery to handheld computers. Surg Endosc 2004;18:997.

[26] Pagani L, Jyrkinen L, Niinimaki J, et al. A portable diagnostic workstation based on a Web pad: implementation and evaluation. J Telemed Telecare 2003; 9:225.

[27] Berguer R, Forkey DL, Smith WD. The effect of laparoscopic instrument working angle on surgeons' upper extremity workload. Surg Endosc 2001;15: 1027.

[28] Berguer R, Rab GT, Abu-Ghaida H, et al. A comparison of surgeons' posture during laparoscopic and open surgical procedures. Surg Endosc 1997; 11:139.

[29] Hemal AK, Srinivas M, Charles AR. Ergonomic problems associated with laparoscopy. J Endourol 2001;15:499.

[30] Nguyen NT, Ho HS, Smith WD, et al. An ergonomic evaluation of surgeons' axial skeletal and upper extremity movements during laparoscopic and open surgery. Am J Surg 2001;182:720.

[31] Herron DM, Gagner M, Kenyon TL, et al. The minimally invasive surgical suite enters the 21st century. A discussion of critical design elements. Surg Endosc 2001;15:415.

[32] Kenyon TA, Urbach DR, Speer JB, et al. Dedicated minimally invasive surgery suites increase operating room efficiency. Surg Endosc 2001;15:1140.

[33] Durrani AF, Preminger GM. Three-dimensional video imaging for endoscopic surgery. Comput Biol Med 1995;25:237.

[34] Hanna G, Cuschieri A. Image display technology and image processing. World J Surg 2001;25:1419.

[35] Herron DM, Lantis JC 2nd, Maykel J, et al. The 3-D monitor and head-mounted display. A quantitative evaluation of advanced laparoscopic viewing technologies. Surg Endosc 1999;13:751.

[36] Hofmeister J, Frank TG, Cuschieri A, et al. Perceptual aspects of two-dimensional and stereoscopic display techniques in endoscopic surgery: review and current problems. Semin Laparosc Surg 2001;8:12.

[37] van Bergen P, Kunert W, Buess GF. The effect of high-definition imaging on surgical task efficiency in minimally invasive surgery: an experimental comparison between three-dimensional imaging and direct vision through a stereoscopic TEM rectoscope. Surg Endosc 2000;14:71.

[38] Chang L, Satava RM, Pellegrini CA, et al. Robotic surgery: identifying the learning curve through objective measurement of skill. Surg Endosc 2003;17:1744.

[39] Dakin GF, Gagner M. Comparison of laparoscopic skills performance between standard instruments and two surgical robotic systems. Surg Endosc 2003;17:574.

[40] Renda A, Vallancien G. Principles and advantages of robotics in urologic surgery. Curr Urol Rep 2003;4:114.

[41] Kuo RL, Delvecchio FC, Preminger GM. Virtual reality: current urologic applications and future developments. J Endourol 2001;15:117.

[42] Preminger GM, Babayan RK, Merril GL, et al. Virtual reality surgical simulation in endoscopic urologic surgery. Stud Health Technol Inform 1996; 29:157.

[43] Shah J, Mackay S, Vale J, et al. Simulation in urology–a role for virtual reality? BJU Int 2001; 88:661.

[44] Matsumoto ED, Hamstra SJ, Radomski SB, et al. The effect of bench model fidelity on endo–urological skills: a randomized controlled study. J Urol 2002;167:1243.

[45] Merril JR, Preminger GM, Babayan RK, et al. Surgical simulation using virtual reality technology: design, implementation and implications. Surg Technol Int 1994;III:53.

[46] Jacomides L, Ogan K, Cadeddu JA, et al. Use of a virtual reality simulator for ureteroscopy training. J Urol 2004;171:320.

[47] Johnson DB, Kondraske GV, Wilhelm DM, et al. Assessment of basic human performance resources

predicts the performance of virtual ureterorenoscopy. J Urol 2004;171:80.

[48] Watterson JD, Beiko DT, Kuan JK, et al. Randomized prospective blinded study validating acquisition of ureteroscopy skills using computer-based virtual reality endo–urological simulator. J Urol 2002;168:1928.

[49] Wilhelm DM, Ogan K, Roehrborn CG, et al. Assessment of basic endoscopic performance using a virtual reality simulator. J Am Coll Surg 2002; 195:675.

[50] Shah J, Darzi A. Virtual reality flexible cystoscopy: a validation study. BJU Int 2002;90:828.

[51] Adrales GL, Park AE, Chu UB, et al. A valid method of laparoscopic simulation training and competence assessment. J Surg Res 2003;114:156.

[52] Gettman MT, Kondraske GV, Traxer O, et al. Assessment of basic human performance resources predicts operative performance of laparoscopic surgery. J Am Coll Surg 2003;197:489.

[53] Gor M, McCloy R, Stone R, et al. Virtual reality laparoscopic simulator for assessment in gynaecology. BJOG 2003;110:181.

[54] Schijven MP, Jakimowicz J. The learning curve on the Xitact LS 500 laparoscopy simulator: profiles of performance. Surg Endosc 2004;18:121.

[55] McFarlane N, Denstedt J. Imaging and the Internet. J Endourol 2001;15:59.

[56] Kuo RL, Delvecchio FC, Babayan RK, et al. Telemedicine: recent developments and future applications. J Endourol 2001;15:63.

[57] Goldberg MA. Teleradiology and telemedicine. Radiol Clin North Am 1996;34:647.

[58] Crump WJ, Pfeil T. A telemedicine primer. An introduction to the technology and an overview of the literature. Arch Fam Med 1995;4:796.

[59] Takeda H, Minato K, Takahasi T. High quality image oriented telemedicine with multimedia technology. Int J Med Inform 1999;55:23.

[60] Byrne JP, Mughal MM. Telementoring as an adjunct to training and competence-based assessment in laparoscopic cholecystectomy. Surg Endosc 2000;14:1159.

[61] Janetschek G, Bartsch G, Kavoussi LR. Transcontinental interactive laparoscopic telesurgery between the United States and Europe. J Urol 1998; 160:1413.

[62] Lee BR, Bishoff JT, Janetschek G, et al. A novel method of surgical instruction: international telementoring. World J Urol 1998;16:367.

[63] Lee BR, Caddedu JA, Janetschek G. International surgical telemonitoring: our initial experience. In: Westwood JD, Hoffman HM, Stedney D, et al, editors. Medicine meets virtual reality: art, science, technology: healthcare (r)evolution. Amsterdam (the Netherlands): IOS Press; 1998. p. 41.

[64] Moore RG, Adams JB, Partin AW, et al. Telementoring of laparoscopic procedures: initial clinical experience. Surg Endosc 1996;10:107.

[65] Rosser JC Jr, Herman B, Giammaria LE. Telementoring. Semin Laparosc Surg 2003;10:209.

[66] Micali S, Vespasiani G, Finazzi-Agro E, et al. Feasibility of telesurgery between Baltimore, USA and Rome, Italy: the first five cases. J Endourol 2000; 14:493–6.

[67] Lee BR, Png DJ, Liew L, et al. Laparoscopic telesurgery between the United States and Singapore. Ann Acad Med Singapore 2000;29:665.

[68] Link RE, Schulam PG, Kavoussi LR. Telesurgery. Remote monitoring and assistance during laparoscopy. Urol Clin North Am 2001;28:177.

ELSEVIER
SAUNDERS

Urol Clin N Am 33 (2006) 409–423

UROLOGIC
CLINICS
of North America

Pediatric Urologic Imaging

Lane S. Palmer, MD[a,b,*]

[a]Division of Pediatric Urology, Schneider Children's Hospital of the North Shore-Long Island
Jewish Health System, New Hyde Park, NY, USA
[b]Departments of Urology and Pediatrics, Albert Einstein College of Medicine, Bronx, NY, USA

There have been significant advances made over the past decade in imaging the genitourinary tract in children. Ultrasound, voiding cystourethrography (VCUG), and diuretic renography currently dominate the radiographic imaging of children with urologic complaints or anomalies. Prenatal diagnosis of urologic anomalies has improved with advances in ultrasound technology [1]. The use of ^{99m}Tc-mercaptoacetyl glycyl^3 (MAG$_3$), greater uniformity in performing the diuretic renography [2], and SPECT imaging have improved the diagnostic quality of nuclear imaging.

Improvements in CT and MRI now offer better adjunctive studies and in some cases a definitive study. Spiral CT has improved imaging for stone disease and tumor staging because of its rapidity and reduction in motion artifact and the need for sedation. Finally, MRI continues to grow as an imaging study for complex anomalies but also may have a role in evaluating obstruction and infection [3–5]. In this article, the discussion will focus on ultrasound, VCUG, and nuclear studies; however, the other imaging modalities will be discussed when pertinent.

Imaging modalities in children

Ultrasound

Ultrasound is the most commonly performed study of the urinary tract. It is performed routinely prenatally as a screening tool for congenital anomalies, the first study performed following

urinary tract infections [6], and the primary study of the acute scrotum in many institutions [7]. When evaluating the urinary tract, the study should include the kidneys and the bladder. Ultrasound images of the kidneys are taken in longitudinal and transverse views assessing renal length (well-established nomograms exist [8]), degree of hydronephrosis (using the Society for Fetal Urology grading system [9]), renal scarring (although nuclear studies and MRI are more sensitive), and the presence of duplication anomalies, cystic renal disease, and dilation of the proximal ureter. Bladder ultrasound assesses bladder volume and the efficacy of bladder emptying and the presence of ureteroceles, bladder masses, dilated distal ureters, or other abnormalities of the pelvis. Testicular ultrasound with Doppler is user-dependent and requires probe placement over the painful area; however, it avoids radiation, is readily available, assesses symmetry and architecture, and carries sensitivity and specificity similar to nuclear scintigraphy that previously was the standard study for evaluating the acute scrotum.

Contrast voiding cystourethrography

The second most common study in pediatric urology is the VCUG. When properly performed, the contrast VCUG provides an excellent view of the anatomy and some sense of function of the bladder and urethra. The plain film taken before catheterization may detect sacral or bony abnormalities, spinal dysraphism, and abnormal bowel gas patterns suggestive of a mass effect. Once catheterization is established and contrast is instilled, an early anteroposterior film will visualize a ureterocele or bladder tumor best. To evaluate

* 1999 Marcus Avenue, M 18, Lake Success, NY 11042, USA

E-mail address: lpalmer@nshs.edu.

urologic.theclinics.com

for vesicoureteral reflux, steep oblique images are then taken of the bladder and renal fossae just before voiding and again during voiding. The bladder images also assess bladder emptying and urethral anomalies. The urethral catheter need not be removed during voiding. Post void films complete the study [10].

Nuclear imaging

Kidney

The static renal scan assesses cortical abnormalities such as infection and scarring using ^{99m}Tc-dimercaptosuccinyl acid (DMSA). The diuretic renogram involves intravenous injection of a radiotracer that is reabsorbed by the tubules (MAG$_3$ or DTPA), timely injection of a diuretic (furosemide, 1 mg/kg), and bladder catheterization. Hydration (oral or intravenous) before injection prevents artificially poor tracer uptake. Differential renal function is measured in the first 2 minutes after initial injection. The reduced background activity seen with MAG$_3$ has led to its preference over DTPA at many institutions. Finally, tracer drainage from the collecting system is assessed after timely injection of furosemide (typically at the peak of tracer uptake or at 20 minutes after injection of the tracer). The time needed for drainage of 50% of the tracer correlates with the obstructive state of the kidney.

Bladder

Radionuclide cystography provides some of the information described for contrast VCU with less exposure to ionizing radiation but without providing adequate anatomic detail. The tracer is instilled into the bladder, and the appearance of tracer in the area of the renal fossa is evaluated. The presence of reflux is graded as mild, moderate, and severe. The role of radionuclide cystography is more limited than contrast VCUG.

Scrotum

99mTc-pertechnetate is injected intravenously, and blood flow to the testes is evaluated immediately and by delayed images.

Renal anomalies

Hydronephrosis

Renal pelvic dilation is the most common ultrasound abnormality of the kidney seen on prenatal or postnatal ultrasound [11]. In the prenatal period, dilation of the renal pelvis in the anteroposterior dimension is measured in millimeters, with the risk of a significant uropathy increasing with the time of detection [12] or size of the pelvis [13]. In the postnatal period, dilation is divided into broader grades such as the system offered by the Society for Fetal Urology (Fig. 1). In the highest grade, renal parenchymal thinning will be seen. Hydronephrosis needs to be distinguished from the normal renal pyramids. The pyramids are small noncommunicating hypoechoic ovoid or round structures that are distributed radially around the kidney. They have no relation to hydronephrosis, so they will remain present in the face of a dilated renal pelvis.

Hydronephrosis may be primary and either obstructive or nonobstructive; or it may be secondary to other processes, many of which are described in this article. Thus, VCUG is indicated to assess for vesicoureteral reflux or other pathology. Diuretic renography is performed to determine obstruction and differential renal function. Some authors advocate for the MRI reporting comparable functional and drainage information to nuclear scintigraphy but with an anatomic image without radiation [4,5].

Renal cystic diseases (Fig. 2)

Multi-cystic dysplastic kidney

The characteristic findings on ultrasound are of multiple cysts of variable size that do not communicate and a paucity of renal parenchyma. The noncentral location of the largest cyst helps to distinguish the multi-cystic dysplastic kidney (MCDK) from the severely hydronephrotic kidney. Notwithstanding this difference, it can be very difficult to distinguish between the two entities. Documenting the lack of function by nuclear scintigraphy using either DMSA or MAG$_3$ may help to make the distinction. CT or MRI may improve the imaging of the nature of the parenchyma between the cysts. The cysts of a MCDK often involute, and the renal unit contracts or disappears; this phenomenon can be followed by ultrasound. Abnormalities may be found in roughly 40% of the contralateral kidneys such as duplication, hydronephrosis, and obstruction on ultrasound. Because vesicoureteral reflux also can be seen into the stump of the MCDK or in the contralateral kidney, a VCUG is indicated [14].

Autosomal recessive polycystic kidney disease

The diagnosis of autosomal recessive polycystic kidney disease is made easily on ultrasound.

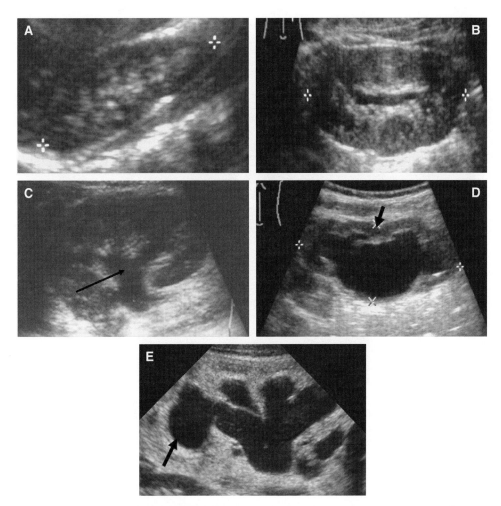

Fig. 1. Renal ultrasound images corresponding to the grades of hydronephrosis according to the Society for Fetal Urology grading system: (*A*) 0-none; (*B*) 1-mild pelvic dilation; (*C*) 2-moderate pelvic dilation (*arrow*); (*D*) 3-dilation including calyces, normal parenchyma (*arrow*); (*E*) 4-calyceal dilation and parenchymal thinning (*arrow*).

Both kidneys are extremely large, reniform, homogeneous, and hyperechoic. The hyperechoic appearance stems from the return of sound waves from numerous interfaces created by the ectatic dilated renal tubules.

Autosomal dominant polycystic kidney disease

This entity consists of bilateral multiple renal cysts of variable size on ultrasound. Early in the course of the disease, cysts are fewer in number and the renal parenchyma relatively normal with respect to corticomedullary differentiation and echogenicity. The cysts tend to grow with time compressing the renal parenchyma as the patients are followed with serial ultrasounds. When the cysts are large enough, there may be distortion or compression of the renal pelvis. Hemorrhage into a cyst is imaged best by CT or MRI.

Unilateral renal agenesis

Unilateral renal agenesis can be suspected on plain film on which bowel occupies the renal fossa. Otherwise, the diagnosis is suspected by an empty renal fossa on ultrasound. The diagnosis needs to be confined by DMSA, MRI, or CT where no functioning renal tissue is found in the abdomen and pelvis (or rarely, the chest). VCUG, either contrast or radionuclide, is indicated because of the high incidence of associated vesicoureteral reflux [15].

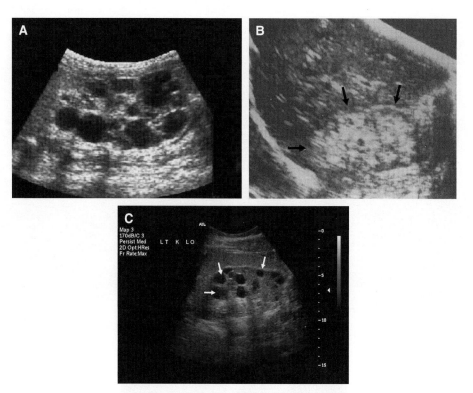

Fig. 2. Renal ultrasound of cystic disease. (*A*) Multi-cystic dysplastic kidney (MCDK) with cysts of variable size with the largest cyst noncentrally located. (*B*) Autosomal-recessive polycystic kidney disease (ARPCDK) in neonate with large very echogenic kidney (*arrow*). (*C*) Autosomal-dominant polycystic kidney disease (ADPCDK) in child with variable cysts (*arrows*), adequate parenchyma.

Renal ectopia

The location of the kidney outside of the renal fossa can be found on ultrasound, IVU, CT, or MRI. The fused ectopic kidney can be found by ultrasound, but CT or MRI allow for better imaging of the malrotation. The horseshoe kidney (Fig. 3) can be suspected by ultrasound in which both kidneys are positioned caudal to their usual position and there is evidence of malrotation. Because these kidneys are at risk for uretopelvic junction (UPJ) obstruction, ultrasound will detect hydronephrosis. The isthmus between the two kidneys may have renal function, and this can be evaluated by nuclear scintigraphy (DMSA or MAG$_3$). Serial ultrasounds are performed to screen for Wilms' tumor. A suspected mass is imaged better by CT or MRI.

Ureteropelvic junction obstruction

Hydronephrosis can be detected by ultrasound (Fig. 4), CT, MRI (Fig. 5), or IVU. Most cases are detected by ultrasound either prenatally or after a urinary tract infection. This will be used as a starting point to discuss the Society of Fetal Urology grading system. When UPJ obstruction is suspected, the ultrasound demonstrates a centrally located hypoechoic area of considerable size extending and possibly blunting the calyces (grade III). The parenchyma of the kidney may be compressed and thinned compared with the contralateral kidney (grade IV.) When there is intermittent obstruction and flank pain, the grade of hydronephrosis may appear less impressive than expected [16].

Once hydronephrosis is detected by ultrasound, its obstructive nature must be established. The gold standard for this diagnosis remains the diuretic renogram using MAG$_3$ or DTPA. Greater standardization of this study has reduced the confounding variables associated with its interpretation. The study allows the assessment of relative renal function and the washout of the tracer following the administration of furosemide.

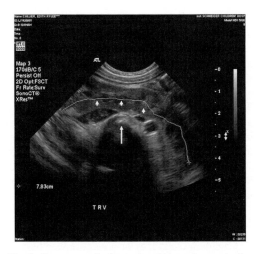

Fig. 3. Sonogram of a horseshoe kidney demonstrating caudal location of malrotated and fused kidneys. Spine (*arrow*), right kidney (*arrowheads*).

In conjunction with appropriate drainage curves, the t ½ value of >20 minutes establishes the presence of obstruction.

In infants and young children, the cause of UPJ obstruction is commonly an intrinsic narrowing of the ureter. In older children, however, as in adults, the presence of blood vessels feeding the lower pole of the kidney may cross anterior to the ureter at a similar location, kinking the ureter and causing symptoms. The presence of crossing vessels is established best by retrograde pyelogram, where a linear filling defect is identified consistently. Direct imaging of the vessels and their course can be accomplished by CT [17] with contrast or by MRI.

Collecting system duplication (Fig. 6)

The presence of a duplicated collecting system is very common [18]. Most children live out their lives without knowledge of this anomaly. Most inconsequential duplications are discovered incidentally on prenatal ultrasound or later in life when abdominal imaging is performed for nonurologic reasons. Duplication, however, can be clinically significant in cases of ureterocele, ectopic ureters, UPJ obstruction, or reflux, all of which are associated with duplication. These duplications also may be discovered during prenatal ultrasound or after the entities have become clinically significant.

Ultrasound must include both renal and bladder images to best document the nature of the duplication. In the simplest case, renal ultrasound identifies two central echogenic foci separated by a bar of renal parenchyma of normal echogenicity, absence of hydronephrosis, and nonvisualization of the proximal ureters. The bladder is normal in thickness, distension, and contour, and the distal ureters are not visible. The situation becomes more complex as the ultrasound identifies hydronephrosis in the upper or lower pole collecting system, dilation and possible tortuosity of the proximal or distal ureters, upper pole scarring or dysplasia (shrunken hyperechoic region), or ureterocele.

The performance of VCUG and diuretic renogram supplements the ultrasound. Vesicoureteral reflux most commonly is associated with the lower pole of the duplication and is graded using the International Grading System [19]. The lower pole is also more likely to sustain a UPJ obstruction, while the upper pole most commonly is associated

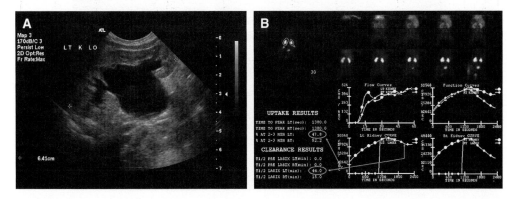

Fig. 4. Child with uretopelvic junction (UPJ) obstruction. (*A*) Ultrasound demonstrates grade three left hydronephrosis and maintenance of parenchyma. (*B*) Diuretic renogram with ^{99m}Tc-mercaptoacetyl glycyl^3 (MAG3) demonstrates adequate differential function and minimal drainage response of the left kidney after the administration of furosemide (*arrows*).

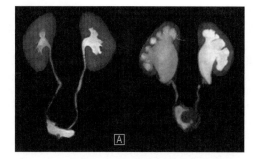

Fig. 5. MR urogram in the T2 phase demonstrating normal renal and ureteral anatomy (*left*) and bilateral ureteral–pelvic obstruction (*right*). (*Courtesy of* Andrew Kirsch, MD)

with obstruction at the distal ureter. The drooping lily is the most notable radiographic sign of an obstructed upper pole duplication, producing the downward and lateral displacement of the lower pole on IVU. Other radiographic signs of duplication include: fewer than expected calyces, particularly of the upper pole, displacement of the ureter away from the tips of the transverse processes, and misalignment of the renal axis along the psoas. The VCUG, when properly performed using a nonballooned catheter, dilute contrast, and the acquisition of early filling voiding images, will identify a ureterocele and any associated reflux; it may intimate or identify the location of an ectopic ureteral orifice when there is reflux during the voiding phase. The washout curves and images from a diuretic renogram can assess obstruction from the lower pole when UPJ obstruction is suspected, or the upper pole when there is ureteral ectopia or an associated ureterocele.

Stones

Calculi in the kidney or ureter are seen best on ultrasound and noncontrast CT (Fig. 7). Ultrasound is useful in detecting medium-sized or large stones. They appear as echogenic foci with posterior shadowing. The shadowing helps to distinguish the stone from fat, or blood vessels. When stones are small, they may be difficult to identify or to determine whether the stone is actually

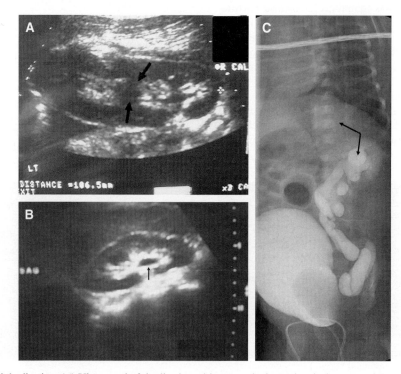

Fig. 6. Renal duplication. (*A*) Ultrasound of duplication without any hydronephrosis demonstrating two central echogenic foci separated by a bar of normal renal parenchyma (*arrow*). (*B*) Duplication with hydronephrosis only of the lower pole (*arrow*). (*C*) Voiding cystourethrogram (VCUG) demonstrates vesicoureteral reflux into the lower pole collecting system without contrast in the upper pole (*arrows*).

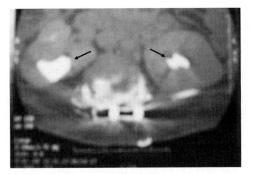

Fig. 7. Noncontrast CT demonstrates large stones in the pelvis of both kidneys (*arrows*).

two smaller stones in close proximity. Hydronephrosis behind the stone often can be seen.

Noncontrast CT using narrow (3 to 5 mm) slices is the most sensitive imaging study for urolithiasis [20]. It accurately assesses stone location, size, number, and associated hydronephrosis. The spiral CT allows for imaging to occur

with speeds that dispense with the need for sedation in children. CT is more useful than ultrasound in documenting bladder stones, especially in the augmented bladder, where small stones may hide among the folds of bowel.

Pyelonephritis

Radiographic signs of pyelonephritis can be seen by all imaging modalities.

The static renal scan is performed using DMSA. This agent binds to the proximal convoluted tubule and therefore assesses cortical abnormalities such as infection and scarring and differential renal function. Images in the anterior, posterior, and oblique views are taken several hours (2 to 4 hours) after intravenous injection of the DMSA (Fig. 8). Differentiation of cortical scarring from acute infection requires DMSA imaging at least 4 months after the last acute infection. MRI has been shown to differentiate cortical scarring from infection by comparing T1 and T2 weighted images obtained before gadolinium injection with T2 weighted images and fast spin echo inversion recovery images following gadolinium injection (Fig. 9) [3]. Ultrasound findings of pyelonephritis include increased renal size and heterogeneous architecture secondary to edema and pelvic dilation, all of which typically resolve after treatment. Contrast CT will demonstrate wedge-shaped segments of low attenuation that radiate to the surface from the collecting

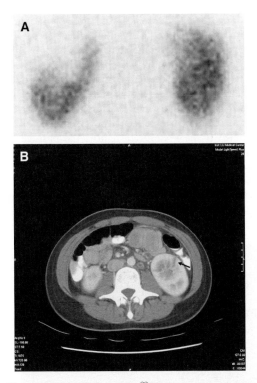

Fig. 8. Pyelonephritis. (*A*) ^{99m}Tc-dimercaptosuccinyl acid (DMSA) scan of child hospitalized with clinical pyelonephritis. In this prone view, note the poor uptake of tracer in the upper pole of the left kidney. (*B*) Wedge-shaped area of left kidney with poor uptake and low attenuation on CT (*arrow*).

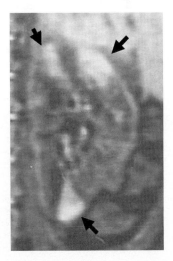

Fig. 9. Pyelonephritis as imaged by MR. This is a T2 weighted image with inversion recovery sequence. There is persistence of signal in the wedge-shaped upper and lower poles of this left kidney (*arrows*).

system. There also will be mild hydronephrosis, enlarged size, and delayed uptake of contrast and transit into the collecting system.

Renal vein thrombosis

Diagnostic imaging of the kidney with suspected renal vein thrombosis is best performed by ultrasound or CT and nuclear scintigraphy. Ultrasound of the kidney during the acute phase will reflect edema with increased renal size and loss of corticomedullary differentiation. The parenchyma is hypoechoic early on but becomes hyperechoic with fibrosis. Thrombi in smaller vessels are seen as radiating linear echogenic bands in the parenchyma. Lack of function is confirmed by nuclear scintigraphy. CT demonstrates enlarged edematous heterogeneous kidneys with poor uptake of contrast. In later phases, atrophy may be documented by all three studies, and calcifications may be seen in the area of the thrombi.

Ureteral anomalies

Megaureter

Megaureter, as indicated by the name, reflects a wide ureter (greater than 7mm). The cause of megaureter has been divided into refluxing, obstructive and nonrefluxing, nonobstructive, or primary megaureter. The radiographic findings associated with each of these categories correlates with the names. Once ultrasound defines the presence of a dilated ureter, the categorization continues with a contrast VCUG looking for dilating vesicoureteral reflux that is congenital or secondary to posterior urethral valves, ureterocele, or functional voiding disorders leading to elevated

bladder pressures. In the absence of reflux, the obstructive nature of the megaureter is evaluated by diuretic renogram ($t\frac{1}{2} > 20$ minutes). If the degree of reflux raises the suspicion of obstruction at the UPJ or the prospect of there being obstruction and reflux, then the radionuclide study is indicated to evaluate for obstruction. If the cause of the obstructive megaureter is not determined by these imaging studies, IVU, MRU [21], or CT can be used to provide greater anatomical detail and reveal the presence of a congenital stricture, ureteral valve, or the location of an ectopic ureteral orifice. In cases of megaureter in which surgery is not indicated or is being held in reserve, the child is followed with serial ultrasound and other studies when indicated. In cases of refluxing megaureter, VCUGs are performed until resolution, either spontaneous or surgical.

Ureterocele

As in other conditions that have been described, the triumvirate of renal and bladder ultrasound, VCUG, and diuretic renography constitutes the radiographic evaluation of the child with a ureterocele. The variable effect of ureteroceles is reflected on the imaging studies (Fig. 10). Bladder ultrasound [22] is effective in diagnosing the presence of the ureterocele, a round, thin-walled, cystic structure of variable size at the bladder base; the dilated ureter leading into this cystic structure often can be seen also. The ureter will be dilated if the ureterocele retards the passage of urine, obstruction at its extreme, or is associated with reflux. The contralateral ureter may be dilated if the ureterocele impinges on the contralateral orifice impairing the passage of urine, undermines the integrity of the antireflux

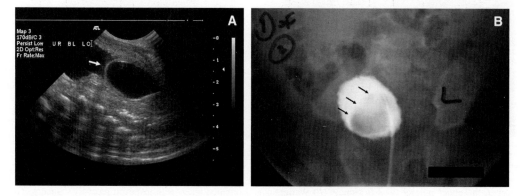

Fig. 10. Ureterocele seen on ultrasound (*A*) as cystic mass along floor of the bladder and by early images of VCUG (*arrow*) (*B*) as filling defect (*arrow*). This VCUG image could be confused with the balloon of a Foley catheter.

mechanism, or obstructs the bladder outlet, causing elevated bladder pressures. This discussion also applies to hydronephrosis seen on ultrasound in the ipsilateral or contralateral kidney to the ureterocele. The other important parameter evaluated by ultrasound is the nature of the collecting system, whether single or duplicated.

VCUG is important for proper documentation of the ureterocele. When suspected by ultrasound, dilute contrast and early imaging can avoid missing the ureterocele by obscuring it with dense contrast or effacement of the ureterocele by bladder distension. The ureterocele appears as a filling defect of variable size within the bladder. The everting ureterocele (Fig. 11) appears to be outside of the bladder and can be confused with a bladder diverticulum [23]. Vesicoureteral reflux may be seen in the ipsilateral lower pole system or the contralateral kidney. VCUG is important postoperatively, especially after cystoscopic puncture, where iatrogenic reflux is the most common complication.

The diuretic renogram will determine the differential renal function and the drainage patterns before and after the administration of furosemide. The regions of interest should separate out each renal moiety. As previously discussed, drainage of one half of the nuclear activity from the system in

over 20 minutes defines the presence of obstruction, while drainage in under 10 minutes defines the absence of obstruction. In the presence of postoperative hydronephrosis, the diuretic renogram is useful in assessing surgical success.

Although IVP is performed less commonly today, there are classic findings of ureteroceles on IVP that should be presented. The cobra head (Fig. 12) or spring onion deformities are seen when the radiolucent wall of the ureterocele surrounds the ureterocele filled with contrast. The drooping lily represents the downward and lateral displacement of the lower pole system by the hydronephrotic obstructed poorly functioning upper pole system.

Bladder anomalies

Vesicoureteral reflux

Vesicoureteral reflux is detected commonly following an abnormal prenatal renal ultrasound or during the evaluation after a urinary tract infection. Ultrasound, prenatal or postnatal, may demonstrate various degrees of hydronephrosis or hydroureteronephrosis. The degree of hydronephrosis does not necessarily correlate with the grade of vesicoureteral reflux [24]. Despite this fact, renal ultrasound often is employed as a screening tool among older siblings of probands with reflux. If there has been scarring associated with reflux and urinary tract infections, the ultrasound is a poor study except in advanced scarring, where an irregular renal contour, loss of corticomedullary differentiation, or a contracted kidney may be seen. The presence of the scars and dysplasia

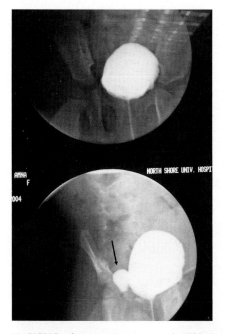

Fig. 11. VCUG of an everting ureterocele. This image was taken late in the VCUG and was confused with a diverticulum (*arrow*). The ureterocele was not seen on the early images of the VCUG.

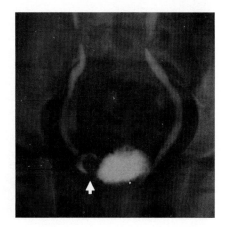

Fig. 12. IVU demonstrating the classic cobra head of a ureterocele (*arrow*).

is documented best by DMSA scan where areas of decreased uptake of tracer will be seen, and significant differences in differential function might be seen.

The demonstration and grading of reflux still is made best by contrast VCUG (Fig. 13). Cyclical VCUG, in which repeated filling and emptying occurs, may increase the sensitivity of the study to detect reflux. Grading is assessed according to the International Reflux Study Grading System (I to V). In addition, assessing the degree of ureteral dilation assists in surgical considerations. The VCUG also allows for the evaluation of bladder and urethral anatomy. Radionuclide VCUG (Fig. 14) is suited best for cases in which anatomic considerations are not at issue, such as after surgery, in follow-up studies of children on prophylactic antibiotics, and in screening of siblings without urologic complaints. The grading of reflux after radionuclide VCUG is less specific (ie, mild, moderate and severe).

Neurogenic bladder

Imaging of the neurogenic bladder is primarily by VCUG and ultrasound. The plain film taken at

the start of VCUG may demonstrate the dysraphism responsible for the child's bladder problem. VCUG will demonstrate bladder trabeculations, sacculations, and diverticulae. In more severe cases, the Christmas tree bladder (Fig. 15) may be characterized by a vertical orientation and multiple diverticulae. Any associated reflux will be documented. Ultrasound will demonstrate bladder wall thickening, associated hydronephrosis, or hydroureteronephrosis caused by reflux or high bladder pressures. Both studies will provide information regarding the postvoid residual and thus the bladder's ability to empty.

Bladder diverticulum

Bladder diverticulae occur in several settings [25]. Congenital out-pouching occurs posteriorly and can grow larger than the bladder. Hutch (paraureteral) diverticulae are congenital, variable in size, and may lead to reflux or prevent its spontaneous resolution. Finally, smaller, multiple diverticulae may reflect high bladder pressures suggestive of bladder outlet obstruction (posterior urethral valves, urethral obstruction, detrusor–sphincter discoordination) or neurogenic bladder

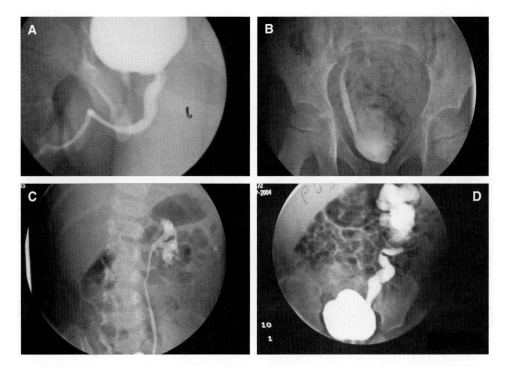

Fig. 13. (*A*) VCUG demonstrates the absence of vesicoureteral reflux in a smooth bladder and normal urethra. International Reflux Study grade 1 (*B*), grade 3 (*C*), and grade 5 (*D*) of reflux are demonstrated.

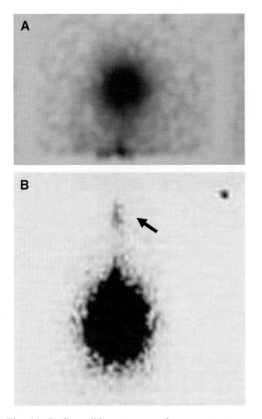

Fig. 14. Radionuclide cystogram demonstrates tracer only of the bladder (*A*) and into the collecting system consistent with moderate reflux (*arrow*) (*B*).

dysfunction. Ultrasound may demonstrate bladder wall thickening but can miss identifying diverticulae unless they are substantially larger. In the largest ones, distinguishing bladder from diverticulum can be challenging. Diverticulae

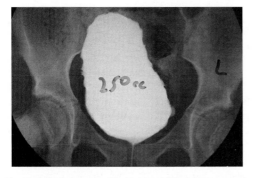

Fig. 15. Christmas tree bladder in child with neurogenic bladder dysfunction from myelomeningocele. The bladder is irregular, elongated in the vertical axis, and studded with diverticulae.

are documented well by VCUG. Bladder trabeculations, small diverticulae, and sacculations may be seen. Hutch diverticulae and the associated reflux will be documented by VCUG. In the case of large diverticulae, anatomical considerations can be made and an assessment of the emptying of the diverticulum (Fig. 16).

Urethral anomalies

Posterior urethral valves (Fig. 17)

To define the effect of posterior urethral valves (PUVs), one needs to employ renal and bladder ultrasound, VCUG, and often nuclear scintigraphy. On ultrasound, hydronephrosis of all grades or hydroureteronephrosis may be seen. If there is renal damage, the ultrasound may demonstrate parenchymal thinning, hyperechoic kidneys and loss of corticomedullary differentiation, or cystic changes. Bladder wall thickening may be seen reflecting detrusor hypertrophy. In the prenatal ultrasound, oligohydramnios can be seen in addition to bilateral hydronephrosis, normal-to-hyperechoic renal echotexture, thick-walled bladder, and a dilated prostatic urethra [26]. The diagnosis of PUV is made by contrast VCUG and is characterized proximally to distally by a relatively narrow bladder neck secondary to bladder neck muscular hypertrophy, dilation and elongation of the posterior urethra, and an abrupt change in caliber at the external sphincter. VCUG also can demonstrate the irregular bladder wall consistent with trabeculations, diverticulae, and bladder wall thickening that occurs in response to the obstruction. Vesicoureteral reflux may be present. Diuretic renography will document the differential renal function and assess urinary drainage. In some cases, bladder wall thickening and elevated bladder pressures will impede the flow of urine to the bladder, and obstruction will be documented by the MAG_3 washout curves. When there are urine collections outside of the kidney secondary to forniceal rupture, ultrasound and CT are excellent imaging studies.

Other urethral anomalies (Fig. 18)

Anterior urethral valve

The anterior urethral valve is a rare anomaly that is often obstructive. It may be found anywhere along the anterior urethra (penoscrotal, bulbar, or penile urethra portions). A contrast VCUG is best at defining the valve's location

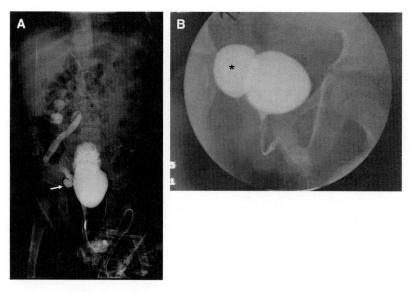

Fig. 16. VCUGs demonstrating (*A*) Hutch, paraureteral bladder diverticulum in child with vesicoureteral reflux (*arrow*); (*B*) a large diverticulum (*asterisk*) similar in size to the native bladder.

and extent and any associated reflux. The valve typically appears as a linear filling defect ventrally with urethral dilation proximally and a narrowing distally or as an abrupt change in caliber. Another appearance is urethral dilation into a smooth bulge within the urethra. When there is obstruction, renal ultrasound may detect hydronephrosis or hydroureteronephrosis.

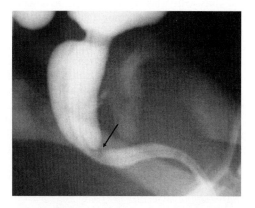

Fig. 17. Neonate with posterior urethral valves confirmed and treated cystoscopically. The ultrasound demonstrates thickened bladder with dilated posterior urethra and bilateral hydroureteronephrosis. The VCUG demonstrates irregular-shaped bladder with dilated posterior urethra and sudden change in caliber at the location of the valve (*arrow*).

Megalourethra

Megalourethra is another rare urethral anomaly best detected by contrast VCUG. The more common scaphoid variant caused by deficiency of corpora spongiosum appears during the voiding phase as boat-like urethral dilation, while the rare fusiform variant caused by deficiency of corpora cavernosum appears as a long floppy dilated urethra.

Urethral duplication

Urethral duplication may be complete or incomplete. A classification system has been proposed that correlates with the findings on VCUG [27].

Urethral diverticulum

The anterior urethral diverticulum forms ventrally along the penile urethra. On contrast VCUG, one sees an oval saccular-shaped collection of contrast along the ventral urethral surface. In some cases, sufficient amount of contrast enters into the diverticulum and may distend enough to compress the urethra and lead to obstruction.

Prostatic utricle

Prostatic utricle is a midline out-pouching emanating from the area of the verumontanum. These are typically small but can be large and

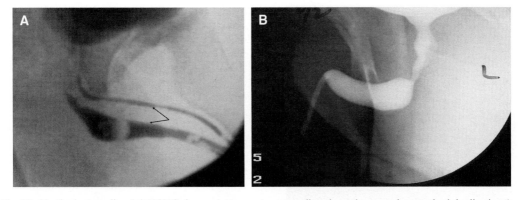

Fig. 18. Urethral anomalies. (*A*) VCUG demonstrates contrast traveling through a complete urethral duplication (*two arrows*). (*B*) Another VCUG demonstrates a saccular type megalourethra.

require more advanced imaging such as CT or MRI to better delineate position.

Cowper's duct cyst

Cowper's duct cysts are also known as syringoceles. There may be out-pouching at the level of the bulbar urethra or a filling defect ventrally on VCUG.

Testicular anomalies

Intersex

The goal of imaging children with ambiguous genitalia is to document the presence or absence of gonads and Müllerian structures. In a palpable gonad, ultrasound may distinguish testicle from ovary by its oval shape, larger size, and the presence of an epididymis. An ovary is more echogenic and may have follicular cysts. Ultrasound is not as reliable as MRI to evaluate the presence or nature of an intra-abdominal gonad. Ultrasound, MRI or genitogram may image Müllerian structures. Pelvic ultrasound may detect the a uterus when it is not a rudimentary structure and otherwise difficult to find. In female pseudohermaphroditism, the uterus can be identified as an oval echogenic structure with fluid in the center along with a prominent endometrial stripe (longitudinal image). Indentation of the vagina by the cervix also may be seen.

The genitogram (Fig. 19) is important, although the role of MRI is growing. The genitogram may document the size and shape of the vagina, the site of confluence between the urogenital sinus and the vagina. It also may identify the cervical impression at the vaginal apex. Patience

and diligence are paramount to performing a high-quality genitogram. The genitogram is performed best by occluding the very distal portion of the urogenital sinus and injecting contrast. As part of a VCUG, retrograde filling of the vagina may occur during the voiding phase, yielding adequate information.

Acute testicular pain

The acute scrotum is assessed best by ultrasound with Doppler or by nuclear scintigraphy. Ultrasound (Fig. 20) will assess the symmetry,

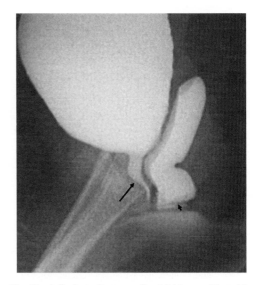

Fig. 19. A flush genitogram of a child born with ambiguous genitalia demonstrating bladder (*arrow*) and vaginal compartments (*arrowhead*).

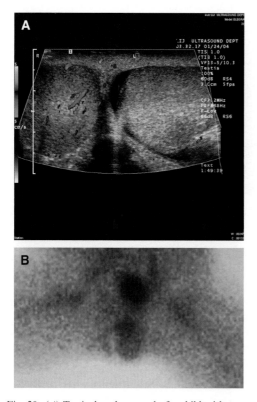

architecture, and perfusion of the testicles in the child who has testicular pain. The nonpainful testis is imaged first and compared with the painful side. Testicular torsion is characterized by a heterogeneous, echogenic testis without flow detectable by Doppler or color flow imaging. The inflamed testis also can have a heterogeneous appearance, but there will be ample flow or hyperperfusion of the testis and epididymis. Reactive hydroceles may be seen in either case.

Nuclear scintigraphy using 99mTc-pertechnetate will assess testicular blood flow to both testes simultaneously (Fig. 21). Ideally, symmetric flow excludes testicular torsion, unless one suspects intermittent torsion. Increased flow to the scrotum is consistent with epididymitis, orchitis, or inflammation secondary to torsion of an appendage. Testicular torsion is suggested by the lack of identifiable blood flow. In cases of missed torsion, there is a hyperemic rim of flow around a central area without tracer uptake.

Summary

Proper imaging of the genitourinary tract is vital to the clinical management of children with urinary or genital complaints. Technological advances continue to improve the quality of the images and reduce the radiation exposure to the child. IVU largely has been replaced by ultrasound, and perhaps MRI will replace CT and even nuclear scintigraphy. The study that is often most vexing to the parents and the child, the VCUG, however, will continue until a new study is devised

Fig. 20. (*A*) Testicular ultrasound of a child with acute testicular pain. Doppler flow is absent on the side of clinical concern for testicular torsion (*arrow*). (*B*) In the second child, there is increased flow consistent with inflammation on nuclear scintigraphy.

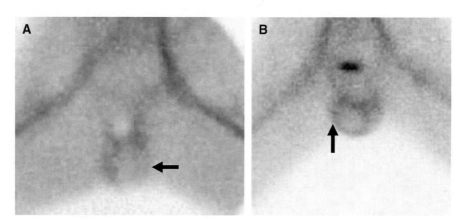

Fig. 21. Nuclear scintigraphy of two cases of testicular torsion. (*A*) There is no scintigraphic activity on the left side (*arrow*) when compared with the right asymptomatic side. (*B*) This study was performed 18 hours after the onset of left testicular pain. There is a rim of flow (*arrow*) surrounding an area without activity consistent with a missed torsion.

that can directly test for reflux and can image the urethra without instrumentation. Nonetheless, the pediatric urologic community continues to benefit from these improvements, allowing for improved patient care.

References

[1] Lebowitz RL. Paediatric urology and uroradiology: changes in the last 25 years. BJU Int 2003;92(Suppl 1):7–9.

[2] Conway JJ, Maizels M. The well-tempered diuretic renogram: a standard method to examine the asymptomatic neonate with hydronephrosis or hydroureteronephrosis. A report from combined meetings of The Society for Fetal Urology and members of The Pediatric Nuclear Medicine Council–The Society of Nuclear Medicine. J Nucl Med 1992;33(11):2047–51.

[3] Weiser AC, Amukele SA, Leonidas JC, et al. The role of gadolinium enhanced magnetic resonance imaging for children with suspected acute pyelonephritis. J Urol 2003;169(6):2308–11.

[4] Jones RA, Perez-Brayfield MR, Kirsch AJ, et al. Renal transit time with MR urography in children. Radiology 2004;233(1):41–50.

[5] Grattan-Smith JD, Perez-Bayfield MR, Jones RA, et al. MR imaging of kidneys: functional evaluation using F-15 perfusion imaging. Pediatr Radiol 2003; 33(5):293–304.

[6] Giorgi LJ Jr, Bratslavsky G, Kogan BA. Febrile urinary tract infections in infants: renal ultrasound remains necessary. J Urol 2005;173(2):568–70.

[7] Siegel MJ. The acute scrotum. Radiol Clin North Am 1997;35(4):959–76.

[8] Rosenbaum DM, Korngold E, Teele RL. Sonographic assessment of renal length in normal children. AJR Am J Roentgenol 1984;142(3):467–9.

[9] Fernbach SK, Maizels M, Conway JJ. Ultrasound grading of hydronephrosis: introduction to the system used by the Society for Fetal Urology. Pediatr Radiol 1993;23(6):478–80.

[10] Fernbach SK, Feinstein KA, Schmidt MB. Pediatric voiding cystourethrography: a pictorial guide. Radiographics 2000;20(1):155–68.

[11] Mandell J, Blyth BR, Peters CA, et al. Structural genitourinary defects detected in utero. Radiology 1991;178(1):193–6.

[12] Ismaili K, Hall M, Donner C, et al. Brussels Free University Perinatal Nephrology study group. Results of systematic screening for minor degrees of fetal renal pelvis dilatation in an unselected population. Am J Obstet Gynecol 2003;188(1):242–6.

[13] Odibo AO, Raab E, Elovitz M, et al. Prenatal mild pyelectasis: evaluating the thresholds of renal pelvic diameter associated with normal postnatal renal function. J Ultrasound Med 2004;23(4):513–7.

[14] Damen-Elias HA, Stoutenbeek PH, Visser GH, et al. Concomitant anomalies in 100 children with unilateral multi-cystic kidney. Ultrasound Obstet Gynecol 2005;25(4):384–8.

[15] Cascio S, Paran S, Puri P. Associated urological anomalies in children with unilateral renal agenesis. J Urol 1999;162:1081–3.

[16] Rooks VJ, Lebowitz RL. Extrinsic ureteropelvic junction obstruction from a crossing renal vessel: demography and imaging. Pediatr Radiol 2001;31(2): 120–4.

[17] Mitsumori A, Yasui K, Akaki S, et al. Evaluation of crossing vessels in patients with ureteropelvic junction obstruction by means of helical CT. Radiographics 2000;20(5):1383–93.

[18] Campbell MF. Anomalies of the ureter. In: Campbell MF, Harrison JH, editors. Urology. 3rd edition. Philadelphia: WB Saunders Company; 1970. p. 1512.

[19] Lebowitz RL, Olbing H, Parkkulainen KV, et al. International system of radiographic grading of vesicoureteric reflux. Pediatr Radiol 1985;15: 105–9.

[20] Palmer JS, Donaher ER, O'Riordan MA, et al. Diagnosis of pediatric urolithiasis: role of ultrasonography and CT scan. J Urol 2005;174:1413–6.

[21] Wille S, von Knobloch R, Klose KJ, et al. Magnetic resonance urography in pediatric urology. Scand J Urol Nephrol 2003;37(1):16–21.

[22] Cremin BJ. A review of the ultrasonic appearances of posterior urethral valve and ureteroceles. Pediatr Radiol 1986;16:357.

[23] Zerin JM, Baker DR, Casale JA. Single-system ureteroceles in infants and children: imaging features. Pediatr Radiol 2000;30:139–46.

[24] Blane CE, DiPietro MA, Zeim JM, et al. Renal sonography is not a reliable screening examination for vesicoureteral reflux. J Urol 1993;150:752–5.

[25] Blane CE, Zerin JM, Bloom DA. Bladder diverticula in children. Radiology 1994;190(3):695–7.

[26] Dinneen MD, Dhillon HK, Ward HC, et al. Antenatal diagnosis of posterior urethral valves. Br J Urol 1993;72(3):364–9.

[27] Effman EL, Lebowitz RL, Colodny AH. Duplication of the urethra. Radiology 1976;119:179–85.

ELSEVIER SAUNDERS

Urol Clin N Am 33 (2006) 425–432

UROLOGIC CLINICS of North America

Index

Note: Page numbers of article titles are in **boldface** type.